Schizophrenia – Who Cares?
A Father's Story

TIM SALMON

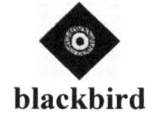

blackbird

Published by Blackbird Digital Books 2015
ISBN: 9780993307027
A CIP catalogue record for this book is available from the British Library
First published in digital-only form in 2013
Copyright Tim Salmon 2013 All rights reserved
Cover artwork c. Adam Grieve, http://adamgrieve.com
All rights reserved. Except in the case of brief quotations quoted in reviews or critical articles, no part of this book may be used or reproduced in any manner whatsoever without written permission from the Publisher.

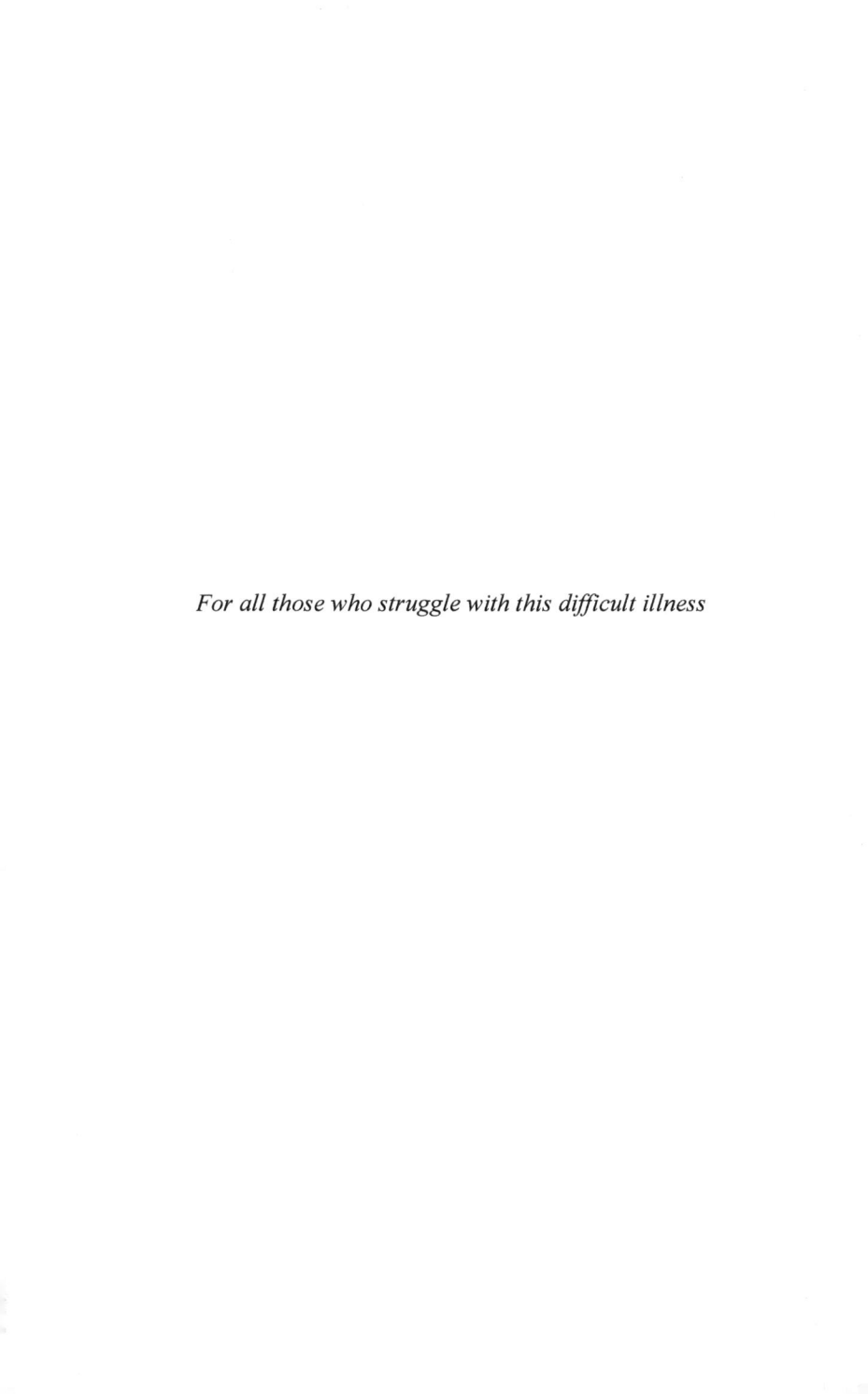

For all those who struggle with this difficult illness

CONTENTS

Prologue 1

Chapter One: Days In The Life Of 7

Chapter Two: The Start Of Things 30

Chapter Three: Learning to Live with It 48

Chapter Four: Care Plan 69

Chapter Five: Living Alone 88

Chapter Six: Contracts and Other Ploys 108

Chapter Seven: Some Calm Before a Storm 124

Chapter Eight: Unsettled Times 137

Chapter Nine: At Last A New Start 154

Chapter Ten: An Unholy Alliance 172

Epilogue 188

About The Author 195

Acknowledgements 196

Reader Resources 197

Prologue

My son got schizophrenia – if it makes any sense to say that anyone 'gets' schizophrenia – some time between 1988, when he graduated from university, and 1990 when he was admitted to hospital as a psychiatric patient for the first time. That is to say that it was during this period that he began to behave in ways that were strange and inexplicable beyond anything I had ever known, beyond anything I had the language to account for. He began to say and do things that appeared to belong in a different, even alien dimension of existence. He began to inhabit a world where I simply could not follow. I tried to keep up: I tried as it were to put my arms around him and protect or save him. He was not gone all of the time, but for much of it I simply could not reach him. I felt as if I had been left behind, baffled and hurt, on some far shore while he lit out into unknowable, desolate regions.

This book is the story of that strange voyage, his illness, as told by and, largely, as experienced by me. I cannot really speak for him for obvious reasons and I have not tried to speak for his mother or his sister, the two other people most affected. Others have played a part too, grieving, succouring, providing sympathy and love: friends, cousins, aunts and uncles; my wife Camilla, my brother Robin and my old friend Geoff in particular.

I have tried to give some idea of what it is like to live with such a tragic illness that typically strikes youngsters in the first full blossoming of their adulthood, blighting their lives like a late frost catching a tree in blossom, preventing its burgeoning fruit from ever setting and coming to maturity: striking them down in those first heady moments when, full of hope and innocent excitement, they reach out for selfhood, for fulfilment, for identity in love and work; and of the isolation, alienation, frustration and abandonment by friends that it brings.

I have also written at some length of the practical frustrations caused by the pitiful inadequacy of the provisions made in our society for looking after people disabled by illnesses of the mind. I have quoted, extensively in places, from the correspondence I have exchanged in the course of these twenty years with various spokesmen of the health and social services. I do not believe that they were malevolent or deliberately unhelpful, but I do think that their almost universal inability to express themselves either clearly or correctly, their penchant for unintelligible jargon, their failure to co-ordinate their activities or even ensure that their own guidelines are followed and their general neglectfulness are shameful and an awful indictment of the nation's education system.

What is schizophrenia, people ask. The short answer is madness: what we used to call madness, loss of reason. Someone who yesterday was quite rational, normal, as we say, is found in the night, naked in the street, distributing pink marzipan piglets to the queues of youngsters waiting to get into a dance hall, making the sign of the Cross and blessing them as if he were the Pope. And that is not much of an exaggeration about the first florid onset of this illness.

What causes it I cannot say. I have not attempted to explain the science of the illness, because I do not know much about it and do not really understand the little I have read. I believe also that not too much is really yet known about its causes, its mechanisms: what exactly goes wrong where to bring about such devastating consequences for those afflicted.

The classic age for the onset of the illness is between eighteen and twenty-five. Usually there is very little warning that anything untoward is about to happen: it strikes, as it seems, out of the blue. There is no way of predicting who is likely to be vulnerable. There is no cure. There are a number of drugs available, discovered by chance, which control, more or less effectively, the most extravagant and melodramatic symptoms, the hallucinations: the hearing of voices, which can impel people to the most drastic of actions like throwing themselves under trains, and the sort of delusional thinking that leads you to believe you are Queen Maeve. They inhibit the production in the brain of the neurotransmitter dopamine which is central to the development of psychotic symptoms. They are however less effective in alleviating the more low-key but in terms of everyday living equally disabling symptoms, like depression, lack of motivation, loss of concentration and memory, a certain dulling of intellectual capacity and paranoid feelings about other people that can transform even routine transactions like shopping into almost unmanageable ordeals.

We used always to hear that the incidence of schizophrenia was pretty much universal, with around one percent of the world's population affected regardless of climate, creed or culture. But this is not true; there are marked variations. For example, city people suffer more than country people, big city people more than small city people, men more than women, migrants more than native populations.

There is a characteristic pattern of symptoms and the illness is diagnosed on this basis. It is a syndrome rather than a single disease which causes pathological changes in people's brains, as many have believed. There is a range of ways in which you can develop these symptoms. The problem as far as curing the illness is concerned is that we do not yet know the pathology of it.

Genes certainly play a role in determining who gets the illness; one or two have already been identified. It seems most likely that the culprits are fifteen to twenty small 'susceptibility' genes rather than a big one that causes the illness. And the variety of schizophrenia that you get – whether you suffer more, for example, from the crazier symptoms like delusions or the more affective ones like depression and lack of motivation – will depend on the hand of genes that birth has dealt you. It is not that the genes cause you to develop schizophrenia, but rather predispose you, make you susceptible to the influence of certain environmental factors.

Among them are difficulties at birth, drug abuse (cocaine, cannabis and amphetamines), growing up in cities and migrating from one country to another. Again it is not that these factors cause the illness but in interaction with genetic susceptibility they can provoke psychotic reactions. Lots of people smoke cannabis regularly and get away with it, but if you belong to the vulnerable minority (around 25% of the population) you could be in trouble. Certainly, among the people I know, many of their schizophrenic sons and daughters smoked a lot of dope in their adolescent years.

"Hearing voices" is the classic symptom. 'Do you hear voices?' is the question patients are asked time and again. The implication always was that you are hearing things which do not exist, which are not there. But an interesting discovery has come about through the development of brain imaging: schizophrenics 'hearing voices' are indeed hearing voices, with the difference, however, that their brains are misinterpreting as coming from external sources sounds which they are really 'hearing' in the part of the brain where we all 'hear' internal speech, as, for example, when silently saying a poem to ourselves. In other words they are not making it up when they say they hear voices; it is rather that their brains are functioning in an abnormal way.

Professor Robin Murray of the Institute of Psychiatry at Kings College in London, the pre-eminent researcher into schizophrenia in this country, said in an interview given to the American Schizophrenia Research Forum in 2005 that he believed schizophrenia was a disease of the mind as much as the brain. 'There is brain dysfunction in schizophrenia, but that dysfunction makes you more vulnerable to particular toxic factors in the social environment. What I find interesting about it is that it is a disorder at the interface between the brain and the social environment. I suspect,' he said, 'some schizophrenic people carry particular susceptibility genes that make them vulnerable to particular environmental phenomena, while other people with schizophrenia do not carry these genes and, therefore, can withstand these particular environmental factors, but are vulnerable to others. That greatly interests me, and I think we're going to be able to identify other such gene-environmental interactions in the next few years.'

Asked whether he thought we would be able to cure schizophrenia, he said, 'I don't think we'll be able to cure it with a single drug. Possibly, a combination of specific pharmacological and psychological interventions tailored differently for different patients may return most people to normal function. Even more excitingly, we may be able to prevent the development of the psychosis. We already have some weakly predictive childhood markers... but we will have more powerful predictors. Will it then be possible to screen such children and carry out neurophysiological or imaging or genetic tests, and identify the children who are especially likely to develop schizophrenia? Will we then be able to intervene before overt symptoms show up?'

There is hope. We must hope. I am sure Prof Murray is right: it is early days. No one has put anything like sufficient money into research into mental illness. How much further on might we be by now if schizophrenia had attracted the funding that cancer has or AIDS?

*

Lastly, I would like this book to be seen as a tribute to the sheer dogged bloody-minded courage and independent spirit of my son. I take my hat off to him.

Chapter One
Days in the Life of...

Until you have lived with it you cannot know what schizophrenia is like. Which is why, at the risk of causing some chronological confusion, I have decided to begin this story *in medias res*: smack in the middle, in plain language! I will go back to its chronological beginning in the next chapter.

In the last few months of my son Jeremy's last hospital admission, when I had decided that I would try to make his story into a book, I kept a diary. I made a record of our conversations, of my thoughts and feelings, and of the various trivial and not so trivial details of our daily lives. I hope this perhaps rather novelistic approach will give some idea of how very odd the oddness of schizophrenia is in the way that it affects how somebody thinks and acts, even when he is relatively well.

Jeremy had been in hospital for eighteen months at this time, not because he was considered too ill to be discharged – that could have happened after six months – but because he was officially homeless. The hostel where he had been living refused to have him back and the "system" had failed to find him anything else. This was the second time in five years that he had had to spend twelve months longer than necessary in hospital. I was in the process of trying to buy a flat for him and we were full of hope that at last we might be able to get him out of hospital and re-established once more in a home of his own.

It was autumn 2006.

*

Sunday September 17th
The phone rings just after six in the morning. Probably Jeremy, I think. As it only rings a couple of times – he often does that,

hanging up before the answer phone kicks in - I stay in bed. About nine I go downstairs to make tea. The light on the answer phone is winking. I press the button to listen: it is Jeremy.

'I feel awful, Dad. Fucking suicidal.'

Damn, I should have answered the phone. His voice is croaky with twenty years of heavy smoking. He sounds frightened. I feel the first reactions of panic myself. My heart tightens, I take a sharp breath.

He seemed perfectly all right yesterday. He has not talked about suicide for ages. What's happened? These thoughts, shadowy in my consciousness, scarcely formed, scarcely needing to be formed: a mix of fear, anxiety and panic, so rehearsed now after nearly twenty years that it has become a reflex. I call his mobile.

'I'm all right now, Dad,' he croaks before I can say anything.

'I just got your message. It gave me a fright. What happened?'

'Oh, I'm sorry, Dad. The f******* woke me up.'

'What, do you mean nurses or...?'

'Oh I don't know. They are just c****'

'I've woken you up again. I'm sorry.'

The phone is already dead; he has rung off, abruptly, as he often does, without a word, without explanation.

Late in the morning he phones again, from his sister's. 'Hi, Dad. I'm feeling chipper. I've had a sandwich and a coffee. I've found Charlotte...'

Charlotte? Who's Charlotte? I think.

'Charlotte Williams. She's a food writer in Belfast.'

'Where are you?'

'I'm over at Sara's.'

'Did you walk?'

He walks miles sometimes; he is frightened of public transport. It is the people; crowds make him uncomfortable. I don't know whether it is fear of what might happen or what people might say or are saying about him: it is a kind of mix of paranoia and agoraphobia.

'I came on the bus,' he said.

That's a good sign, I think: a sign that he is quite well. 'Have you been in touch with Charlotte?'

She was a girlfriend from student days, I remember: twenty years ago now. She ditched him in his last year. People have often asked me if he suffered some shock, some kind of emotional trauma that pushed him over the edge. There is a belief that schizophrenia comes about as a result of a predisposition that is in turn triggered by a shock, like, for a young man, being jilted by a girlfriend. I do not know whether that is true, for my son or anyone else. It seems a rather simplistic explanation to me. Certainly, he was very upset; and it is also true – well attested, indeed – that young men with schizophrenia can become fixated on a particular girl, crossing continents to track her down. I found my son in my car one night, in the days when he used to live with me, when he was first ill. It was two in the morning. 'What are you doing?' I said. 'I'm going to see Charlotte,' he said. 'What, now?' I said, trying to think of persuasive arguments rather than a straight fatherly prohibition against going. 'She's in Belfast and you don't know the way. You haven't got a ticket. Besides, the car isn't insured for you. And what if she is not there? You haven't seen her for two or three years. And I need the car.' Luckily, he got out of the car quite meekly and that was that.

'I heard her voice,' he said.

'Have you actually spoken to her?' I ask, surprised. 'How did you find her?'

The phone has gone dead.

I do not worry. He has been talking about finding Charlotte recently and once asked me to track her on my computer. And the hearing her voice... well, it could be just hearing voices, in the broad sense that he does "hear voices" – the classic symptom of schizophrenia. It could be just his way of saying that she was very present in his thoughts and he had been in a sense communing with her or the idea or memory of her. He does talk like that, in a rather elliptical way, as though certain steps in the process of expressing something were left out, so that his conversation seems to jump in an illogical and, seemingly, "mad" way from one topic to another.

Anyway, he is at his sister's and says he is having a good time. It is a beautiful day. I don't give it another thought.

About two the phone rings again. That will be Jeremy wanting a lift home, I say to my wife, as I go to answer. I don't want to go.

'Dad?'

There is a tired, flat tone to his voice. I am on the alert. We have spoken on the phone several times a day for years; my ear is finely attuned to gauging his mood and state of mind. 'Can you come and get me? I feel shattered. I've had a row with Robert.'

'A bad one?'

'Quite.' My resolve not to fetch him is broken immediately.

'Okay. Where are you?'

'I'm on the corner of Bathurst Road. By the library.

'Okay. Stay there. Don't move. I'll come immediately.'

'I'll have to go,' I say to my wife, who is not his mother. In the twelve years we have been together she has never once shown anything but total sympathy and understanding for my predicament and his, not easy, especially when the person who is the source of such anxiety is not even your own flesh and blood. 'I don't know what has happened.'

The drive to my daughter's takes me past my son's old flat, along streets that I have travelled countless times over the years, my heart in my mouth, an agonising void in my entrails, not knowing what exactly I am going to find, how much damage done, how much grief and pain and bewilderment and sheer bewildering craziness in my son's own state of mind. This time I am only mildly anxious. He has had a row. Well, that is manageable, reparable.

I don't stop at my daughter's but circle the block, forced by the one-way system. No sign of Jeremy by the library. I stop and get out of the car, look up and down the streets. Nothing. Damn, he must have moved. Driven by impatience or by his demons. Now what? I'll go and call on Sara.

I ring the bell, hear steps, but no one comes. Robert and Sara, both of them, appear at the bay window beside the door, looking out rather warily to see who it is. They let me in. 'Oh God,' says my daughter. 'What happened?' 'They had a fight. Jeremy hit Robert and head-butted him.'

'Is he all right?'

Oh God, I think. He is just about to come off his "section". I am trying to get him set up in a flat of his own again. He is on regular medication. And now this. Is he ever going to get better? Is it safe for him to live on his own again?

'How did it happen?' I ask.

Robert understands about mental illness; his own sister killed herself. He is very sympathetic to Jeremy and has handled him well over many years now. I am surprised and disappointed; I have come to rely in a way on the presence of Robert and my daughter, as people who are able and prepared to manage Jeremy and put up with his craziness. At least they are two more people, in addition to his mother and me, who love him and are prepared to maintain relations with him, come what may. It is a relief to know the burden does not fall on me alone. It falls on his mum too, but I feel particularly burdened because I seem to be the one who can manage him best.

Robert, luckily, is not badly hurt: he is bruised and, more than anything, in shock. They both are; they look very tired. 'It was horrible,' my daughter says. 'When Robert tried to hold him, he head-butted him.'

People talk about unacceptable behaviour, setting boundaries... That is all very well when dealing with someone rational. I have learnt a lesson: with the mad, you have to keep the emotional temperature as low as possible. Do not scold or try to reason. When the atmosphere feels stormy - and you certainly learn to recognise the warning signs - back off, keep calm and, if possible, move away from the situation, best of all, physically. Low expressed emotion, high expressed emotion: these are the jargon expressions. Schizophrenics cannot deal safely with a high level of expressed emotion.

I said this to Robert. He was muttering about fighting back and if he did it again.... He was hurt in his male pride as well as being shocked, I know. I said, 'Don't! First, you are dealing with the strength of a madman and you don't know where it might lead. Nothing is to be gained and you might get really badly hurt. You've got to play it down in these situations and, if possible, spot them before they develop and get out of the way.'

Jeremy had been difficult and probably rude. He bombards them with phone calls, sometimes offensive. They often feel besieged by him; it can feel quite menacing. It is different for me. There is not the rivalry between two males of the same age. And Jeremy can be cruel. Robert and my daughter would like to have a baby and cannot. Jeremy has taunted Robert about this. So Robert snapped, understandably, for the first time in several years and told him off. And Jeremy snapped too.

They said they were considering blocking their phone. Sara feels guilty about it. I said, 'You must not feel guilty. You have got to protect yourselves first. If you don't do that, your own lives will be destroyed and you will not be in any position to help him even if you want to.'

It can sound horribly callous: inhuman cruelty, unnatural feelings. I have a friend who put her own son out of the house, knowing that he had no money, no job and nowhere to sleep. It is a terribly hard thing to do, especially for a mother. But she was right. He was making life hell for the rest of the family and she still had one school-age boy at home. Why, you might ask, did not she get in touch with the social services or the mental health teams? For one thing, it was in the middle of the unprepared Thatcherite Care-in-the-Community reforms; and, for another, what makes you think that the "system" can be relied upon to help when you need it? We will come to that later.

I left my daughter's and set off home, wondering if I would find Jeremy somewhere along the way. I did, right by the library where he had said he would be. Hidden by some steps, I had not seen him. He had been waiting an hour.

He got into the car. 'Are you okay?' He looked all right, I was relieved to see.

'I'm tired. You got here first.'

'What do you mean? I could not see you. I looked all round. I thought you had probably gone without me.'

'It was you or the ambulance.'

He said he had been into the corner shop, told the shopkeeper he was schizophrenic and asked him to call an ambulance, which apparently he had done. For a moment I thought perhaps I should go back and call and try to cancel the ambulance, but thought better of it. Had he really called an ambulance? How long ago?

I said, 'I stopped at Sara's when I could not find you. They said you had a fight with Robert. What on earth did you do that for? You know, you must not ever do that, ever, ever. No matter what happens, you must not resort to violence, either verbal or physical. Just go, just get away from the place when you feel things are getting out of hand. When you get in that new flat, you must not take against the neighbours. Just don't have anything to do with them.'

'Of course there will be neighbours. I have to see them.'

'Just promise me one thing. That you will always take your medication without fail. And say sorry to Robert. Write him a note if you don't want to speak to him.'

That is enough of a sermon, I tell myself, and say no more. Does it do any good? We drive past his old flat. I make no reference to it, neither does he.

That is where our present ills began, with the old flat. Well, in a sense. They really began with the onset of the illness. But the present cycle of difficulties, practical difficulties, began there. He threatened a neighbour and the police were called. He had been five years without a hospital admission then. That was in 2001. Since then he has been in and out continually, twice for more than a year at a time. He has never been able to return to the flat; the threatened neighbour is still there and anyway, as a kind and sympathetic other neighbour explained, they would all band together to prevent his return. Unpleasant and hurtful to hear, but can you blame them? In fact I have just sold the flat. That is the money I am going to use to buy him a new one.

Can he manage it? Is he well enough to live on his own? Robert thinks he isn't, but Robert is under shock. Perhaps he is right: that is what many people would say. But what am I to do? What is to become of him? I don't actually think he is any less well than he used to be. Was he able to live on his own then? He did, for better or worse, with fag butts all over the house, strange wavy cultures growing in the sink. He did not starve and he did not burn the house down. He will live like this again, most probably, and his mother and I will have to go in and clean up and help out as best we can. As long as we can avoid trouble with the neighbours...

Monday September 18th

We have coffee quite early at his favourite café on Southend Green. We sit outside, not just because it is sunny. I don't think he ever goes inside, perhaps sometimes in a pub, where it is more spacious. He does not like to feel confined or too close to other people. Girls go by on the street. 'She's pretty,' he says of one. And he gets excited about the prospect of having his own flat again and the girls he is going to have round.

I hope so for his sake. I feel so sorry for him. He has often talked of babies. He will refer to some girl as "the mother of my children": it may be someone he fancies on the ward or a girl he has seen in the street whose name he does not even know. And why wouldn't he long for a girl and for children of his own? But, my God, what a nightmare! How could he look after them? I have a friend whose daughter has had two or three babies taken from her because she was too ill to care for them. But the yearning... This damned illness does not even allow you to have a girlfriend, or only rarely and briefly. He is still a handsome man when he is well, but which of these lovely nubile girls going by in the sun, with their brown shoulders and bellies showing, going to their normal jobs, their normal activities in their normal world, which of them would have him, could have him? But the illness does not lessen the desire for the flesh or the longings for nest and family.

It is a cruel, cruel illness and this perhaps is the cruellest aspect of it, that it unravels your existing relationships and makes new ones all but impossible. Which of his childhood or university friends is still in touch with him or has shown any desire to stand by him in his troubles? There have been one or two, but it is not an impressive record. And why should they, you might say? They had their own young lives to build, families of young children to raise and defend. And who knows anything of schizophrenia, of madness and mental illness, unless they have been there themselves, seen it at close quarters? The awful loneliness. I remember once when I was visiting my son in hospital a girl came up to me, thinking I was a new patient. She was a pretty girl aged about thirty, with a huge scar on her neck and shoulder (was it a burn?) and asked my name. 'I'm not a patient,' I told her. 'I am Jeremy's dad.' 'He is so lucky,' she said wistfully, 'I wish I had a father.'

While we are sitting there in the sun and Jeremy has just ordered a second cappuccino, he stands up suddenly. 'I think I've had enough now. I'd better go, Dad.' And he leaves me.

Later in the day he phones to say, 'Pray for me and Charlotte.' What is he talking about? I wonder. 'Have you been in touch with her?' He has been using the ward computer a bit in Occupational Therapy and downloaded an article about her: she is working on a magazine in Belfast. 'I heard her voice,' he says. 'I'd better go now.'

Wednesday September 20th

It's his fortieth birthday tomorrow. I am a bit anxious about how it will go because of Sunday's fight. It would have been nice to have everyone united, but Jeremy himself seems well. His eyes are clear and his gaze steady, not staring. His brow is unclouded too, the skin stretched normally, not drawn tight as it is when he is not well. He phones only three or four times, even not at all some days. When he is not well, he can phone twenty times and when you pick up the phone there is no one there. Conversations are relaxed and normal. His first call is usually around ten o'clock and he will ask me how I am and what my plans for the day are. Then he will tell me what he has been doing, what sort of a night he has had. Usually he has already been to his café and had a cappuccino. 'It's my regular, Dad. This morning the waitress brought me a cappuccino as soon as I sat down. I did not even have to order it. I like that,' he says with a chuckle. Sometimes he has been up to the Heath already, to sit on one of his benches. He chooses one as far away from other people as possible. Sometimes he has bought a brioche or a sandwich, which he eats out there in the middle of the grass, with a bottle of orange juice.

It is no good worrying about what he eats. Sometimes he eats at the hospital, sometimes he orders take-away. Sometimes he does not eat. I wish he would not drink. On the whole, I don't think he has more than a couple of cans, even when he says he has had too much. He'll have his first beer on an empty stomach in the morning. It is probably not a good thing in combination with the medication. The consultant says it is not. I try not to comment, but find it hard not to say, 'Well, mind you don't have too much.'

What's a couple of cans by many drinkers' standards? And what else is he to do, poor lad? All day for nigh on twenty years with nothing to do, no imposed pattern to his life. What does he do? He reads, sits, writes the thousands of jottings that he calls his work, does what he calls meditation, gets bored, passes time.

I try not to think of those things too much, the lack of a pattern and purpose, the irregularity of his habits, the absence of friends, a life wasted... but you simply must not go down that road. It leads to tears and despair. He manages; he is still there, still putting up resistance; he has not turned into a drug-drowsy zombie as seems to happen to some. He can still explain a complicated scientific notion in clear, rational, succinct terms. He still buys and reads the *Scientific American*.

It is my boy and I love him. There are times when I am filled with fear and despair. When things have seemed to be going well and you start to entertain high hopes that perhaps he will after all make a steady recovery and be able to lead a more "normal" life, suddenly it all goes wrong again. Just when we are on the point of getting him out of hospital, and I have gone off on one of my journeys – I am a travel writer – I phone or his mother phones to tell me that he has just been 'sectioned' again or there has been some kind of fracas on the ward: someone has hit him or he has hit someone. Hardly surprising given the confinement in close proximity of so many people with such intractable and incompatible problems. And my heart sinks, again. Will we never reach a state of equilibrium?

Forty tomorrow...

I have been thinking of what to get him as a suitable present for reaching the significant age of forty. I thought of a laptop, but I am not certain that he will actually use it. I have decided on a nice flat screen telly. If his habits in the old flat are anything to go by, he'll leave the telly on, silent, for company or, who knows, perhaps as a sort of firewall against other intrusions. So, I think, we'll get him a new one as a vital piece of furniture. But there is no point in actually getting it until we have the flat. But we must have something for tomorrow; I'll make him a cake, the richest chocolate cake in my repertoire!

Thursday September 21st

It is the most beautiful day. Bright, blue, clear, warm. A perfect fortieth birthday. I call and wish him Happy Birthday. He sounds happy enough. It is ward round day and the hospital has asked me to attend. So we have a date for 12.30.

I go up on my bike. They let me into the ward. It is locked, always, for security – both ways, I guess: to keep some out as well as some in. Jeremy can come and go as he does because he is deemed well enough to be "on leave," as they call it, for much of the day. Even so you have to have a member of staff let you out and then in again, so no illusions about being really free.

All the staff on duty today are black. This is often the case. White faces are rare on mental health wards, at least below the rank of doctor. Sometimes that makes me angry. How can someone from Ghana or Mauritius or Nigeria build any kind of relationship of trust with someone like my son, university-educated, heir to many generations of educated and artistic people? What do they have in common? Why should he confide in them, talk through his problems with them? And yet we hear endlessly about catering to the special needs of minorities.

Today the two women who let me in to the ward, nurses, I assume, are sweet and charming and full of smiles. And I think to myself that I should not be so critical.

The ward round, as usual, is running late. A nurse shows me to my son's room. 'Sit down, Dad,' he says, 'not too close. I'm meditating.' He has got his legs up on the bed in the lotus position. I can't do that.

We chat for a while. We are going to go down to his mum's. He wants us all to be together for his birthday. That has long been a problem for him. 'If you and mum were together, then I wouldn't be schizophrenic.' It is usually a sign that he is not very well when he begins to talk like this. But he did say that he would like us all to get together for his birthday.

'Do you think we should go and see what time they expect to call us?'

'I'll go, Dad,' he says.

I sit on the end of the bed and wait. This is a new ward; it was opened in July 2005.

When Jeremy returns he is brandishing a ten-pound note. 'One down,' he announces. 'Maggie paid me back.'

He is always acting as banker on his ward, lending money open-handedly. In the past he has lent as much as £200 and, of course, never got it back. I used to worry that he was perhaps being threatened. He may have been sometimes, but as he seems to handle the situation without undue stress I have given up worrying. He has only his Income Support and Disability Living Allowance, like everybody else but he has always managed his financial affairs sensibly, even saving money, although the system does not approve, rather meanly, in my opinion, docking your allowances if you save more than £3000.

We go into the ward round. Today there are only five people in addition to ourselves: the consultant, who runs the show and, in theory, has the final say in Jeremy's treatment and "care package"; a pretty doctor assistant, whom Jeremy rather fancies and who is in charge of the daily detail of supervising his treatment in hospital; a woman whose job is to liaise between the various agencies supposed to be helping him; a ward nurse and another party whose function is not clear. Today everyone is white. Indeed they usually are at this level; it is the nurses and assistants who tend to be black. Often there are as many as fifteen people, various kinds of staff as well as students, which, it is not hard to imagine, can be very intimidating, especially when you are not feeling well. Jeremy can be difficult then, either refusing to attend at all or getting angry and walking out. Sometimes he can be quite funny. At one ward round I attended the consultant was sporting a new moustache. Jeremy walked up to him in front of several other staff and students, looked at him in appraisal, then shook his head and said, 'No, Phil, no. Doesn't suit you.' The consultant, whom I like and trust, just laughed and said something like 'I'm sorry to hear that.'

Today, he is quite calm and relaxed. The consultant asks how he is and I say it is his fortieth birthday. Everyone wishes him Happy Birthday and one of the girls says he does not look it, which pleases him. The consultant brings up the matter of his accommodation and the failure of the system to find him anything. He knows I am trying to buy a flat and I tell him where we have got to. He explains to Jeremy that when it comes to discharge they want to do it gradually. Since he has been in hospital so long, it may take a bit of adjustment going back to civilian life. So they plan to let him go over to the flat and spend some time there during the day for a while and then maybe spend a night and come back to the hospital, so that he can adjust gradually.

Jeremy seems to accept that without resistance, but then he says, 'I have got to have work. Someone has got to find me a job.' And he becomes quite insistent about this. I try to deflect his insistence, by saying that he will be able to get on with his writing.

It is never clear, when he talks about work, quite what it is that he means. No one wants to tell him he could not possibly get a job. I say, well, there are many ways of occupying yourself, working, in effect, without actually being employed, like your writing and reading. And we manage to guide the conversation away from this rather fruitless discussion. The fact is, he is pretty well at the moment, lucid and funny and intelligent about many things, but this insistence about work is a reminder that in some strange way his thinking processes just don't quite work properly, logically.

Today the whole meeting passes in a cheerful, civilised manner and Jeremy and I leave together, Jeremy shaking hands all round. I bike home to fetch the cake and the car and arrange to meet him on the street. We go down to his mum's, which is only a few minutes' drive away. We have some cake. I've brought four candles, one for each decade, and Jeremy blows them out, with some difficulty: his puff has been weakened by twenty years of heavy smoking.

Jeremy says, 'Why can't we all spend some time together?'

'When's Sara coming round?' I say, trying to change the subject.

It is twenty-seven years since I parted from my children's mother. I have never been able to work out exactly what Jeremy is thinking when he says this: is it simply a desire to return to a time before he was ill and the remembered harmonies of childhood? The odd thing is I don't remember him ever saying in the years that intervened between my departure and the onset of his illness that he wished his mother and I would get together again. It has certainly been a regular refrain since. Perhaps it is part of the strange un-realism that is such a characteristic of schizophrenia. It is embarrassing always, I admit, for it plays on my guilt. As there is yet no convincing scientific account of how the illness comes about, no matter how much you try to rationalise, it is hard to exonerate yourself completely: maybe it was something I did... that fear gnaws always at your conscience.

I had hoped Sara would be there, so we could have all been together for a little while. I was afraid the fight might have put her off, but she is nothing if not loyal, no matter how difficult her brother is. Knowing that she is coming I go home, happy that the day has passed off so well.

About five the phone rings. It is Jeremy. 'Can you come and get me? I'm at Mum's.' Immediately – I can't help it – I think, 'Oh Lord, what's happened?' But nothing has happened; he just wants a lift home. 'Shall we meet up and have a coffee or something?'

'OK. Give me half an hour. I'll call you in half an hour.'

When I do call there is no reply, so I call his mum. 'Will you come and get him?' she says. Obviously there has been no communication. 'That is what I'm phoning about. He asked me to come and get him, but he does not answer his phone.' She goes to fetch him. 'He is not here,' she says. 'He must have gone out. He has been out three times already.' She is agitated. 'Well, I am coming anyway,' I say. 'If you see him, keep him there. Tell him I am on my way.'

When I arrive, my ex opens the door. Jeremy has not appeared yet. 'He has been out three times already,' she tells me again. Her voice is agitated, as if something worrying is happening. But she is always anxious. Ever since Jeremy first became ill, she has been in a state of nervous agitation. There has been good cause, you might say, for a mother to be agitated when faced by such an illness in her child. I don't know, obviously, exactly how their relationship is. I know that Jeremy always talks of missing his mum when she is away and of feeling more secure when she is at home. It is of course his childhood home. But he is more difficult with her; she complains that he shouts at her and is abusive.

He is a big man and alarming when angry and she is of a nervous disposition. Somehow this does not help. So often she has called me, 'Will you come and get him? He is being so difficult.' And when I get there I do not find him especially agitated or irrational or even drunk, as she so often claims. But even when he is well, she finds it hard to acknowledge and enjoy. There is always a reservation, a readiness to look on the dark side and, Lord knows, I cannot be accused of extravagant optimism myself. These family histories and differences of personality make the situation so much harder to deal with.

Jeremy shows up shortly after I arrive. His blue eyes are clear; there is perhaps a little tautness in his face, but he seems quite calm to me. He had just been for a bit of a walk, he said. He has changed his mind about coffee; he just wants to go back to the hospital. He is tired. I think the day has probably been quite emotional enough.

He phones me later to say he has had a good day and he loves me. 'Well, I love you too,' I say. He has got much better at saying these things recently. In fact he says it quite often. And he asks after my wife too. These are all good signs.

Wednesday September 27th
He phoned me a little while ago to say that he had some news, 95% good, 5% bad. I thought, 'Oh Lord, what now?' He said, 'Whenever I try to seek help from women, the fair sex, females, the boys always put me down, including you.' I said, 'What do you mean? What sort of help? Has something happened?' He said, 'Well, you know, they don't like it.' I said, 'Are you thinking of any particular incident?' He said, 'My knees crunched.' I said, 'What's the connection? I don't think there is a connection

between your knees crunching and...' And he put the phone down!

There is a history of knees crunching and joints cracking, ever since he was first ill, though Heaven knows what it means. But even allowing for that! What on earth goes on in his poor mind? What strange dislocations, jumps, and this at a time when in many respects he is quite normal! A very odd illness.

Radio 4's *Thought for the Day* has a piece by a clergyman, who talks about Michael Stone or rather a newly produced report on his case. He seems to be representing mental illness as a struggle between good and evil: as if the "goodness" of the young mother and her children who were his victims were somehow an intolerable challenge to the evil in Stone, as if he were tormented by the contemplation of their "goodness". I don't think this is a very helpful way of looking at mental illness. People who are mentally ill can sometimes do terrible things, but it is not because they are intrinsically evil: it is because something has destroyed the capacity of their minds to perceive the world in the terms we regard as normal. I am surprised that a man of God should take this view and write to say so: no reply, of course.

The bishop ended his talk by describing how while visiting Rampton or some other secure hospital he had met an old woman coming to visit her son, as she had done every fortnight for many years. He cited this as an example of the power of love, which it is of course, but it is not uncommon. I know several people – mothers, most often – who have devoted their lives to looking after a crazy and difficult child at home. Some are broken by it, reduced to weary anxiety; others show extraordinary fortitude and good humour.

Friday September 29th

The *Today* programme carried a report on the deficiencies in the mental health services, in the course of which we were told that one in four people will suffer from mental health problems this year. This is not a helpful statistic in my opinion; and it must derive from a definition of "mental health problem" so all-encompassing as to be almost meaningless. It does nothing to draw attention to the plight of the seriously mentally ill.

Saturday September 30th
Jeremy phones early but leaves no message. I dial the 1-4-7-1 callback code which confirms it is him. I call back. He's a bit sleepy. 'Are you at your desk?' 'That's good,' he says, when I tell him yes. 'What are you up to?' 'Well, I'm clean.' 'What do you mean?' 'I've done the laundry, shaved and had a bath.' 'That's a good thing.' 'I'm going to have to slow down now.' 'Okay, I'll talk to you later.'

We go for a short walk in the afternoon, to the Heath, and as usual get no further than one of the benches in the open grassy area above the ponds. It comes on to rain, heavily. I have got one of those wide golfing umbrellas which both protects and in a sense cocoons us. Everyone quickly scurries for shelter leaving us, knees drawn in beneath our cover, isolated in the middle of the grass and the rain. 'I really enjoy sitting here. I feel so comfortable, especially with you, Dad.' I do, too. It is almost as if nothing had ever gone wrong. No before, no after: if only I could keep it like this...

It is so difficult not to think "If only..." In moments like this it is so close to being all right. Couldn't it be? Can't they just...? Surely, there must be some way of... But there is not and you just have to accept, not let your hopes be raised too far nor yet taken from you altogether: when it is good, enjoy it, so that when more difficult times come again you are a little re-charged and better able to resist once more.

Monday October 2nd
I try to bring up the matter of saying sorry to Robert, by letter, if doing it over the phone or face to face is too hard. But he gets cross and I let the matter drop.

Tuesday October 3rd
He phones to say he has been on-line in the Occupational Therapy group and found a website with thousands of Tae's, the name of his Korean former girlfriend. 'I keep her in my heart of hearts,' he says.

That was a real relationship, that lasted several years...

'I heard a snatch of song and it brought tears to my eyes,' he said.

'Songs, smells… yes, those are the things that ambush us and bring long-forgotten people and events right back into the present,' I said, trying to diffuse the sadness, always wanting to smooth the situation over, remove the pain. Like my mother standing up the dead blackbirds! I tried to change the conversation by talking about landlines and mobiles and broadband deals for when he moves into his flat. He does not want to talk about it. 'Dad, you make me tired. I had a good day yesterday,' he adds. 'I ate quite a lot.'

Wednesday October 4th
He calls in the morning to say he is having a cup of tea, but it is not really going down. 'I might go for a croissant, but it is not really worth it.'

He phones again later to say he is having a drink in the garden at the Freemasons. There is no one else there. 'I need a companion with my first drink. With the second I don't want anyone. There was this woman Wendy, who is in the women's ward, hanging around on the landing. She was probably looking for someone to go out with.'

'Attractive?' I ask, hoping always there might be girlfriend material around.

'She has a quite attractive face and upper torso, but she does roll-ups. People who do roll-ups, as you probably know, are a bit…'

'You do roll-ups,' I say.

'But it would be nice to get my leg over… Okay, better go now. Love you, Dad. Thanks for talking to me.'

Sunday October 8th
We meet at Southend Green. He is already there, sitting on a bench in the newly refurbished fountain area. He does not look any different from any of the other people sitting there, a little more isolated perhaps: there is something peculiarly solitary about the solitude of tramps or people with mental illness. He has been on the Heath, 'But it did not go very well.' He explains that

there was a Chinese man. 'He was talking and then he coughed and that gave me schizophrenia.'

Coughs, like cracking knees, have longed played a part in this illness. I can't really understand the significance of them and generally don't ask for an explanation.

Tuesday October 10th
He is already at home when I get in from my run about 9am. He is reading, with the radio on, as usual so low it is scarcely audible. He looks well, no tautness today. He wants to sit in my study while I write, *i.e.* sitting behind me. Well, I like seeing him, but his presence makes it hard for me to concentrate, especially when I am writing about him.

When I come down from my shower he reads me what he has been writing, all he is going to do for the day, he says. There is a quite lucid comparison of some of the Houellebecq novels he has read and a bit about searching for Tae on the internet. Then, before I have to worry about having him sitting behind me while I work, he goes. 'I have to go and buy some salad with Marjorie at Budgen's.'

I don't know who Marjorie is but I assume it is part of Occupational Therapy. Anyway it sounds a sensible project and it is quite an achievement if she has persuaded Jeremy to accompany her. He phones later to say that he has got the ingredients and is on his way back to the hospital but doesn't like tuna and is not going to bother going to the session where the salad actually gets made. Which seems a pity, but does not really surprise me.

He phones again shortly after. This time he is quite agitated, eff-ing and blinding about those f****g... I assume it is the others on the ward, but I have no idea what has been happening. He is also cross because his Ethiopian friend is supposed to be with him but isn't. 'He's a bit soft. It's tiring...' is all I can get out of him. 'We had a conversation about wanking and he said he had never done it. I don't know that I believe him. It's all right, Dad. Don't worry. I'm all right now.' And he rings off.

Wednesday October 11th
He phones to say he would like to look at some of my writing to see how you get it to flow. He says his is all bits, just a sentence or two and he doesn't know how to go on.

We talk about the flat. He says he is worried about the neighbours and hearing voices. I say, 'But if you can tell yourself it's not the neighbours when you hear voices, if you don't associate the neighbours with the voices...' He says he can't help it if he can't see the neighbours' faces and say, 'Oi, John...' But I don't really understand what he means, how the mechanics of hearing voices works. 'But they are going to give me talking therapy and that will help.' He repeats this several times.

This is an encouraging development, though experience suggests it would be as well to be wary; for there has always been a large gap between what he says when he is rational and what actually happens. Still, he has never before been positive about the possibility of help. I make encouraging noises about cognitive behaviour therapy, which I assume is what they are proposing: as I understand it, it is a practical approach to practical problems. Maybe they can help him devise a strategy for neutralising the voices, making them less disturbing.

Thursday October 12th
Jeremy phones about ten. I tell him I'm out of action until after two, because I have to do some writing now and then I've got a Turkish lesson; why don't we meet later. He sounds very croaky. When I ask what he's been doing, he says he went out for half an hour about seven-thirty and then went back to bed for a couple of hours.

The doorbell rings not long after this conversation. Notwithstanding my remark about being busy, it is him. I can't turn him away. He makes a cup of coffee while I make him a couple of bits of toast, which he eats, which is gratifying: I am a great believer in affection through eating. He opens the garden door and sits in the morning sun. 'Go back to work, Dad,' he says, to stop me hovering. I try to but can't really concentrate; he seems a little brooding this morning and I hover, trying to read his mood. The familiar seesaw: hope and anxiety, optimism and anxiety.

He does not stay long and seems more smiley and relaxed than when he arrived. 'It is a pity you don't have a bigger garden,' he says. 'With a lawn.'

He calls me around 9pm, later than usual. 'I just talked to Robin (his uncle). He is so intelligent. He has enlightened me. He just knows what to say.' Then he says he is troubled by voices. He says he keeps hearing 'I would, I would.' 'What does that mean?' I ask. He says it could mean, 'I would kill myself or I would... nothing at all.' And he chuckles at that. 'No, I mustn't mention the dreaded s-word,' he says. I say, 'Can't you just tell yourself it's a voice saying "I would, I would," for whatever reason and sort of file it away, like dumping something in the trash on a computer and then just not pay any attention to it?' He says, 'It's like in Kilburn (where his old flat was). I kept hearing ersatz.'

Then he said he was feeling sleepy. 'I go to bed on the dot at ten o'clock. I love bed. It is the place where everything, where all good things happen.'

'Have you eaten?'

'I had a great big pizza.'

'You eat quite well really, don't you?' I say, seeking to reassure myself.

'Oh yes, I have two square meals a day on average.'

I feel better. 'Good night. Sleep well then.'

'Lots of love, Dad.'

Friday October 13th
I'm waking early these days worrying about the flat. It has been four months now and still we have not exchanged contracts. What is the vendor up to? Is he going to change his mind? My solicitor says no: he has gone so far, the place is unlet, he won't back out now. I wish I could be confident. I tell her she will have to be optimistic for me. This has happened to us once already this year. The vendor changed his mind, condemning Jeremy to another few months in hospital. Is this one going to do the same? What am I going to say to Jeremy if he does?

Saturday October 14th
I pick Jeremy up in the car. The idea is to go somewhere, but he decides that the Heath is far enough. We leave the car and go and sit on one of his benches in a secluded spot only a hundred metres or so into the park. He is happy and relaxed. He talks again about how his uncle, my brother, seems to understand about hearing voices and his whole situation.

'But you are not supposed to have exclusive relationships,' he adds illogically. That's what they said at the Richmond Fellowship.'

That was years ago now, when he was first ill.

'What on earth did they mean?' I said.

'They meant sexually, I think.'

'There was that rather pretty Italian girl you had your eye on.'

'Francesca,' he said. 'But I like having an exclusive relationship with my old man,' he added. 'I like having my dad to myself.'

I know that, but it is nice when he says it and I love him for it. But we have always been close. It makes it painful to see his condition, but it also makes it easier to deal with because whatever may happen between us – quarrels, rudeness, even violence – that solidarity cannot be broken: I know that any nastiness is short-lived and unintended. The difficult thing about exclusiveness is its exclusiveness: I have a wife and a daughter. My wife is very understanding. I worry that my daughter has felt left out, neglected by me. But perhaps that is my guilt. She too understands the situation and anyway has her own married life. I think others in this situation have the same feelings about their sane children: that they neglect them because they find themselves obliged by the illness to devote so much time to watching over the sick one. And perhaps it is not neglect: it is just that one is preoccupied continuously by the demands of the illness.

'I've got to have some water,' Jeremy decides suddenly. These urges are irresistible imperatives. There can be no negotiation. We leave our bench to go up to the fountain in the lime avenue. Then, suddenly it is too far: he wants to go to the one by the car park.

'That's no walk at all,' I say. I prevail on him to walk as far as the limes. When we get there all he wants is a swallow and a spit. 'But you didn't even drink anything,' I say and realise there is no point in pursuing the matter.

As we are walking back, he says, 'My schizophrenia, the illness, I can feel it like this. It sort of comes up and over my head.' He makes a gesture, running his hand up his nape, over the top of his head and down over his eyes. I do not understand. He says, 'Do you remember when you first admitted me my legs were stiff, I couldn't bend them?' I don't remember. But what on earth is the origin of this strange theme of stiff or creaking joints?

I say nothing about "when you first admitted me". That too is something which comes up from time to time, as if I had brought the illness about by taking him to hospital. This time he does not accuse me directly, as sometimes he does.

Chapter Two
The Start Of Things

It is almost exactly eighteen years, since the dread word schizophrenia was first mentioned as an explanation of what might be happening to my son. He had been out of university for a year and some odd and unexpected things had been happening.

He was a clever boy. He had won scholarships and academic plaudits all through his school career. At university he wobbled, or so it seems with hindsight, switching courses at the end of his first year.

I had married for a second time by then and was living between Greece and London; my new wife was Greek. I was surprised how upset Jeremy sounded when he phoned me in Athens to tell me he could not go on with chemistry. He had always been good at science and maths, although it was always slightly surprising to me that he had chosen that path, for he seemed such a natural for the humanities. I attributed the strength of his emotion to a youngster's uncertainty and sensitivity.

He changed to a history degree, but rejected the university's advice to start afresh in the first year. It was sensible advice for someone who had done only science for the previous four years. I could not persuade him either. So he started on second year history. Everything seemed to be going along quite normally. I went to Edinburgh to see him. He seemed settled. He had friends. At the end of the year he failed one of his courses and the university told him he would have to retake the exam at the beginning of the next academic year. He went to America, worked as a house-painter and then spent his money hitching round the country. He came back without leaving any time for revision and failed his second attempt at the exam. The university told him he would have to abandon the history Honours course and be content with a medley of third year courses ending in a General Degree. The first setback in his life. Well, certainly the first academic setback. My mother would have said a more important setback was the day I left his mother.

It was a disappointment certainly, but nothing out of the ordinary. He did not seem to be too downcast. And there was certainly nothing odd in his behaviour or demeanour. I thought he looked a little wild and haggard when he came out to Greece for a summer holiday, but that may have been because of the dope he was smoking: a lot, according to his sister. And there may have been some other things; years later he told a psychiatrist he had done a lot of drugs at university. Should I have noticed? Would it have made any difference if I had? And was he doing it because I had caused some terrible wound in leaving his mother when he was thirteen, as my mother would have it?

And then what happened? I find it hard to remember clearly. I was in a state of permanent anxiety about what my wife was planning to do. She had insisted that she needed to be in Greece to do the things she wanted to do in life. Four years had gone by, during which I commuted, anxiously trying to stay a father to my children. My wife had just embarked on a hugely ambitious project to set up a radio station. I was jealous of the people she was involved with; I could see no end to her commitment to living in Greece and feared that she might be going to leave me. I stayed in Greece.

Jeremy returned to London after his Greek holiday and started to look for a job as a trainee accountant: a choice that I found out of character and inexplicable. Like a good, understanding modern father – in contrast to the fathers of the Greek boys I had been teaching who, without hesitation, decided what their sons were going to do with their lives – I decided that if this was my son's choice, then I would support him. But to my astonishment he drew a blank wherever he tried. He had a degree; he was good at maths. Yet none of the big firms would even consider him. Through a childhood friend I arranged for him to go and talk to a once famous athlete and well established accountant. He reported that interviewing Jeremy was like talking to the living dead.

Was I alarmed already? A comment like that coming from someone with a reputation for sympathy and openness and good works with young people did frighten me. I was anxious. Parents are anxious when things do not seem to be going right for their children. Here was my son, who had been sociable, liked, successful, a good athlete, clever, adventurous, being compared to "the living dead". Finding accountancy an odd choice myself, I had thought that perhaps the people who were interviewing him also sensed that he was forcing himself, that he was not really cut out to be an accountant. But "living dead" as a sober assessment, that struck a chill into me. That seemed to suggest something more sinister than mere indifference or unsuitability to a career or poor interviewing skills. I guess I was frightened already. For you know as a parent, you do not have to be told: your sixth sense has already picked up the undertone of threat, of danger and risk, before it has matured, before it has emerged as a nameable disaster. I could not yet name it, I did not know; yet the cold had entered my heart. I lived with a sense of dread, of foreboding.

I do not remember the exact sequence of events nor my own movements that winter of 1988-9. Jeremy was living at his mother's. At some point he did get a job, not on a prestigious training course, but in a lowly capacity with a local firm of accountants in Maida Vale. He put on his suit and went to work. He phoned me at lunch-time on the second day, in tears; he did not want to go back, he could not do the tasks his employer set him. I offered to pick him and bring him home for lunch. He did not want to do that. He went back to work. I do not even remember whether he completed the week. It turned out that the task he could not do and so frightened him was sorting letters, into two piles.

I just felt desperately sorry for him. I had no idea what was happening. I did not know how to comfort him, how to help him in any way. And it must have been terrible for his mother too; she bore the full brunt of it as he was living in her house. But I could not discuss the situation with her. All she had ever said about anything to do with the children since the day I left her was that the situation was impossible: Jeremy was impossible, everything was impossible. I had been gone ten years by this time.

I went back to Greece to try to patch things up with my wife, whose radio project had ended in catastrophe. We drove up to Paris for the celebration of the bicentenary of the French Revolution. Jeremy came to meet us, staying with some French relatives; his mother, who is French, had grown up in Paris. We spent a couple of days together. He used to get on well with his Greek stepmother and we had quite a happy time in spite of my anxiety.

While he returned to London, we set out to drive back to Greece, stopping for a couple of days with French cousins near Marseille. There was bad news. Jeremy had started work in a local bike shop in London; he had long been interested in cycling. But he had lost the job, in the first week.

My wife went on alone to Greece. I flew back to London, leaving the car with our cousins – both psychiatrists, as it happens, one of whose son has since also developed schizophrenia.

I do not remember what I did or what Jeremy did. I did not know what to do. Jeremy asked if he could use my garage to set up a little business doing bicycle repairs. He had some cards printed and started to advertise. He got one or two customers. I like cycling too. I had no problem with my son becoming a bicycle expert. He got himself taken on as a cycle courier as well. He took part in some cross-country mountain bike events and organised some rides on Hampstead Heath. Healthy physical activity, out of doors: must be a good thing. I thought these were hopeful signs, even if he did seem rather strange and his relations with his friends seemed to be unravelling.

I returned to Marseille, picked up the car and drove it to Greece. With my wife I went to the little island where we had a house. There was the usual round of dinners on the quayside with friends, including some new ones my wife had picked up. They had various artistic pretensions; she had decided that she too was really an artist. There was talk about telepathy and the occult, subjects that seemed quite of character for my normally rationalist wife. Though we were physically in the same place and superficially relations were normal, it felt as if moorings had been cast; strange tides and currents were swirling about. I did not feel at all safe. A glamorous friend showed up from Crete where she lived on a boat with her husband; they were going to sail to Tunisia and needed an extra hand. My wife encouraged me to go. Out on the real sea I did momentarily feel safe, away from land, outside the world in a kind of limbo, half in love with the glamorous friend who, I knew, was also in the throes of marital problems. On my return I went back to the island. My wife stayed in Athens. She would come later, she said. Days went by and she did not come. Then suddenly she came, for the weekend, bringing dozens of potted plants, in flower, from a nursery she had passed on the way. They were ready-mades, the kind of the thing you plant out in a municipal garden when the display needs changing: not my idea of gardening and I said so. That set a sour note for the weekend. She left again.

In the week that followed, it must have been in the first days of October, Geoff, one of my closest friends, phoned from London. 'I think you had better come,' he said. 'Jeremy is being very strange. He bit Dolly's finger the other day.' This was the friend who was looking after our London house in our absence. I told my wife, who said she would come as soon as she could.

I told David, an old friend and neighbour, who has now spent most of his life in Greece. We ate and drank and got maudlin together in the evening. I told him I had a premonition that I would not be returning to Greece, at least not in the same circumstances as before. He said he would come down to the ferry with me in the morning.

Morning came. The quay was wet and smelt of salt. The wind had got up in the night and the narrow channel separating us from the mainland was very choppy. We waited a while and word went round that the ferry could not sail, or rather could not dock if it did. I waited two days, anxious and restless, for the wind to drop. I could have gone if it had not been for the car; the water taxis were running.

David came with me once more. We said goodbye. He waved for a few minutes and walked back along the quay. I remember standing on the open ferry deck, looking back at the gentle rounded profile of the island's interior rising behind the pink-tiled roofs, palm trees and bright white houses of the waterfront as the rusty old ship widened the gap of water between us. I felt heavy and sad. That little voice in my head persisted. I knew I would not be coming back; something had ended, though I did not yet dare to give it its full name. I suppose it is not too melodramatic to say that life was never to be the same again.

*

In London I found my son white-faced and strained. His skin seemed drawn tight across his forehead and his brow stood out in an unnatural angry ridge. His eyes had a wide blank look. He was working as a bicycle courier. He would ring me up sometimes, in tears, to tell me that he had ridden all the way to Tower Hill to pick up a package for delivery in Shepherds Bush, but when he got to Shepherds Bush he found he had forgotten the package.

Frightening times: this clever, talented boy, unable suddenly even to pick up and deliver parcels reliably. He obviously found it frightening too, though would not talk about it. He kept harping on my divorce from his mother, on our no longer being together: as if somehow, if we came together again, his problems would be resolved, he would somehow be joined up again, reunited with himself. It was a line of argument which played havoc with my sense of guilt, that lingering doubt – still lingering doubt – that if I had not gone when I did, then none of this might have happened.

We went to family therapy, all of us together. I suppose there was talk about divorce and its consequences. I remember the therapist accusing me of being "too maternal". I am not sure what she meant by that, unless it was that I tried to be too involved, to cocoon my children, to fuss round them. But I felt, I had always felt, that if I did not see to the practical matters, nobody would. How can you speak openly in front of your children about differences that remain unresolved, still, after fifteen years of marriage and ten of separation?

I found a certain comfort in these weekly meetings. The therapist advised us to continue beyond the initial two-or-three-session trial run. 'She would, wouldn't she?' was my ex's comment. 'She wants to build a new swimming pool.' My ex's main concern seemed to be to shift as much blame as possible for everything on to me: Jeremy's anger and general out-ofcontrolness as a schoolboy, various practical difficulties – all this had come about since I left the home and of course as a consequence of it.

Ten days or so after my return to London my mother phoned to say my father had had a stroke. I leapt in the car and set off home, begging him not to die before I got there. He survived, although never really left his armchair again. My Greek wife, throughout this time, kept saying she was going to come, but did not.

One day Jeremy entered a mountain bike race somewhere in east London. We went together, with his bike in the car. It was a beautiful autumn day, I remember. I watched him race, round and round a rough track with its pits and jumps, hoping somehow that he could re-find himself, become himself again through this kind of activity. But his physical form was not what it had been either. He fell behind and then, I think, the gears or the chain broke and he had to retire: another blow in a growing catalogue of setbacks and failures. I felt so sad for him and sick at heart myself.

A friend, wanting to give him some work, asked him to wallpaper her bathroom. He had never hung wallpaper before and put the strips on crooked; they bubbled as they dried and I had to re-do it.

It must have been around this time that I switched on the TV one evening to find myself in the middle of a play about a young man who had begun to behave very oddly. There was an uncanny resemblance between the things he did and said and my son's behaviour. The word schizophrenia was mentioned. I did not have a very clear idea of what it described, but I remember the fascination and the dread with which I watched this fictional boy going mad.

Finally my wife arrived, a few days before Christmas. I do not remember what I felt. I was full of fear, fear about how things stood with her, fear for my son, fear for my father. I do not know what was going through my wife's head. At times she seemed tender; at other times she seemed different from the person I had known, as if she had had a personality change: her views about the world seemed to have changed, so that I found myself in disagreement with her about things we had always formerly agreed about. A friend – a former teaching colleague – was staying, invited by my wife. Later I wondered whether she had invited him deliberately, knowing what was going to happen. I found his presence inhibiting; I could not talk, discuss anything with my wife.

Jeremy had conceived the idea of joining a cycling trip to Morocco in February or March. My wife encouraged me to go with him. A few days after Christmas, on a gloomy afternoon, I set off on a bike ride by way of getting into training. I rode along the disused railway track that begins at Crouch Hill. On the way back, as I was approaching Kenwood, a car shot out of Stormont Road without stopping. I was going fast. I braked as hard as I dared and swerved, just avoiding a collision. I had to stop and wait a few moments to recover from the shock. Every time I ride past, which I often do, I am reminded of that fateful day.

When I got home, the teacher friend, Geoff and my wife were sitting in the kitchen. I said a breezy hello and sat down. My wife went upstairs, returned a few minutes later and asked, 'Where's my suitcase?' I said, 'Why? Are you going?' 'Yes,' she said, announcing her intention to all three of us, so that my friends learnt of her departure at the same time as me. I went upstairs with her and asked again, 'Are you really going? Just like that?' And she left.

The leaving was a complicated, shilly-shallying business that dragged on for months. Well, in a sense. In my head, perhaps. But she never spent another night in this house. I was beside myself.

As sorrows come not single spies, in the midst of this chaos the main drains blocked, threatening to flood the living room with liquid shit. Teams of emergency plumbers came and sat with legs dangling in the curious sump in the middle of my living room floor – a left-over from the days when the house was a garage – cracking their macabre professional jokes while their pumps sucked out the muck. Yet every time it was emptied, within days it was full again. I appealed to the Council, who diagnosed a collapsed connection to the public sewer and started digging a mine-shaft in the street. The work lasted for weeks. The bill came to several thousand pounds and the insurance company refused to pay, finding, as they always do, some specious reason why my particular case was not covered by their policy; they would not accept the Council engineer's account of what had caused the problem. I think it was two years before I finally got the money out of them and then only because, coming home one day, I happened to catch the end of a television programme about insurance companies which ended with the address and phone number of an insurance ombudsman. It was the threat of the ombudsman that finally persuaded them.

And no sooner had we got the drains flowing sweetly once more, when the great white domes of mushrooms appeared between the treads on my stairs: dry rot. The house filled with the din of pneumatic drills digging up the floor, the stairs were cut out: for two or three weeks I had to clamber up a step-ladder balanced on a pile of cement bags in order to get to bed.

I persuaded Geoff to come and live with me. He was homeless and on his own and our two histories had been closely intertwined for six or seven years already. I could not sleep. I started smoking for the first time in fifteen years. I had no appetite. Geoff and I would stay up late, drinking and smoking and playing the guitar, him pretty well, me very amateurishly. He was extraordinarily patient, while I droned on night after night about my lost Greek wife, and I guess he did his share of talking too, for he had been left by his long-time girlfriend. One night we brought Peter Starstedt, who had written the hit song *Where have you gone to, my lovely*, home and he and Geoff jammed until the small hours. We had met him in a local spaghetti bar, alone and rather forlorn. I did not know who he was but Geoff did and they started talking music.

Then one morning Jeremy's mother phoned to say that he had attacked her: at least, he had climbed into her bed during the night and bitten her. This was clearly some kind of crisis: something had to be done. Who can know what was going on in his poor tormented mind? His mother was frightened. His GP said he was suffering from a delayed adolescent crisis, which struck me as about as improbable an explanation as you could find.

That something was terribly wrong was obvious, but what? There is nothing more frightening than not knowing, not having a name to describe this terrifying and mystifying experience. I rang my son's GP; he refused to see me on the grounds of medical confidentiality. I was furious.

I went to see a doctor friend. He said the situation sounded serious and gave me the name of an old and well-respected Viennese psychiatrist friend of his who was still working as a consultant at the Charter Nightingale clinic. We arranged an appointment and he asked me to type up a couple of pages describing what had been happening and send it to him before our appointment.

I went to see him with dread in my heart. He said at once that on the basis of what I had written it seemed very probable that my son's problem was indeed schizophrenia. What is it? I wanted to ask. How do you get it? What can you do about it? He said I should try to get a referral from the GP for my son to go in for an assessment with a psychiatrist.

I phoned and made an appointment to see the GP as if I were my son. I waited with some apprehension in the surgery waiting-room in case anyone recognised me from the days when I too was one of their patients. When my son's name was called and I went in, the doctor was clearly taken aback. I explained what I had done and why. He tried to throw me out. I told him I was not going to leave and said that I thought his diagnosis of my son's condition as a delayed adolescent crisis was preposterous given the way he was behaving. I told him I had been to see a psychiatrist who thought it was probably schizophrenia and that he ought to have a referral for an assessment and that he had recommended the Royal Free, which, as it happened, was, indeed still is, our local hospital. It was an ill-tempered meeting, but the doctor at least agreed to make the referral.

Jeremy came to live with me. The atmosphere was tense. He was often strained and upset. He was still working as a cycle courier; he had a job with the *Sunday Correspondent*. He often complained about a particular woman receptionist he got his commissions from. With the wisdom of hindsight I think much of what he reported was probably taking place in his own head: I suspect now that many of the exchanges he reported as being with her were actually voices heard in his head – his voices. For this is now a long established pattern: an obsession with a particular person, whom he often refers to as saying things to him, being in some way responsible for what he feels and experiences. I tried to offer advice, explain away any unpleasantness, trying to reassure him that I was sure she did not mean anything unkind and maybe if he could think about her like this, then he would not be so troubled.

Sometimes he would fly off the handle completely, in a mad, wild rage, his face white with fury, and I did not know what I had done or said to upset him. More than once I thought he was going to hit me. Geoff told me that no matter how hurtful or how crazy anything Jeremy said or did was I should always remember that it was his illness, not him, doing or saying these things. That was probably the single most helpful piece of advice I have ever received regarding Jeremy's illness. Geoff had watched his girlfriend's brother go round the same bend; he had become obsessed with a Greek girl, would climb drainpipes to get into her flat and then wreck it; he had gone all the way to Athens to do so on one occasion.

I was hurt and bewildered and afraid and it did indeed seem to me that my son had become someone I did not recognise and could not communicate with any more, could not get through to: that is how it appeared – as a matter of getting through some barrier, getting through some fog of I-did-not-know-what to make contact once more with the person I had known as my son. And I was frightened for myself: desperately lonely and shaken by my wife's departure for reasons I did not really understand and frightened about my future. I had no income; I had given up teaching, my profession, ten years before. I signed on briefly, then got a couple of hours work a week standing in for a teacher in a language school in Golders Green who was away on maternity leave. My mother did not help: never one to contain her own anxiety she wrote me letters referring to Geoff, Jeremy and myself as a pathetic trio, which made us all furious!

Jeremy went off to Morocco on his cycling trip. I don't know how he got there, how he managed it, but he did. He organised his tickets, packed his bike, joined up with his little group and – miracle of miracles – came back in one piece. Some of the group, I think, must have been very understanding. His mother was worried sick. So was I, but I thought then and have continued to think that, no matter how alarming they may seem, it is good for his sense of himself to take some risks, to do some of the things that he would certainly have done if he had never fallen ill, although I confess that some years later, when he was planning a trip to Thailand during a period of not being at all well, I contacted the airline he was planning to book with and warned them not to sell him a ticket. He was proud of himself for having managed the Morocco trip and wrote an article about it that was published in the *Bicycle* magazine. It was well written. He could have written, indeed might well have made that his career if things had not gone so drastically wrong.

He tried to keep up his connections with some of his fellow cyclists. I got the impression that they were not too keen, which obviously hurt him. But his relations with everybody had become so strange, fraught with all sorts of difficulty. His way of looking at the world, his comments, his way of talking about things had become so strange that people who did not know him must have been alarmed. That was one of the most distressing things: you watch your own loved and talented child suddenly being shunned by the world, unable to get a toe-hold anywhere and, while you can see clearly that he is ill, he himself will not accept it. An impasse.

How did I cope? I do not really know. I started going to psychotherapy with a wise old lady who had lived a bohemian, adventurous life herself. I became very dependent on my weekly visits; in fact, I think I went twice a week for a while. And I went for a run most mornings, either on Hampstead Heath or Primrose Hill. I started going more often to Primrose Hill because I had noticed a pretty blonde woman who walked her dog most days at the same time as my run. After a week or two I plucked up courage and found some pretext for talking to her. She was married and lived somewhere nearby. We walked and talked. And thereafter every time my run coincided with her walk, a coincidence I tried to bring about as often as possible, I would fall in with her. She had a sister who suffered from similar troubles to my son's but had recovered sufficiently to be able to manage some kind of independent life, which was encouraging. She was obviously well off and led a life quite different from mine, with a holiday home in the Bahamas. But she was warm and pretty and ready to talk and, I sensed, probably not too happy in her marriage. I fantasised about having an affair with her but she never gave the slightest hint that that was what she wanted, so I contented myself with these twenty or thirty minute walks as often as I could get them.

The Greek wife went to America. I only ever saw her again a couple of times after that. I tried to persuade Jeremy that he ought to go and have a psychiatric assessment and to my surprise he agreed. We went up to the Royal Free together and he was seen by a woman psychiatrist, in Out Patients, it must have been. She seemed kind and gentle and understanding. I was not able to talk to her but after she had seen Jeremy she said she would like him to come in for a week for observation. He seemed amenable.

I guess it was only a few days later that we packed his Moroccan hold-all and drove to Friern Barnet. I have never been so frightened in my life as when we turned into the drive at Friern Hospital. I do not know what I had been expecting but it was not that. And God knows how Jeremy felt. We turned between the lodge gates. The tarmac of the drive had a worn uncared-for look. The wide lawns before the house had been gang-mowed but not very recently. We drove up to the house, an enormous Victorian pile. I forget whether it had a tower and turrets. They would not have been out of place. It looked like a cross between a castle and a dungeon, grim and severe and run-down. It was a bin, an old-fashioned lunatic asylum. We parked the car and got out. I do not know what Jeremy was thinking. I do not remember if we spoke, if I tried to be jolly and put a bright face on it. I know that I felt leaden: utter leaden despair, as if my son were about to be incarcerated for ever. We went to reception, a reasonably well-appointed hall just inside the main door. I gave our name and we were directed to Six Oaks ward. I think someone accompanied us. It was on the ground floor.

We followed an immensely long corridor walled in solid Victorian brick painted, like the old 1870 schools, with layers of shiny cream paint. We passed through heavy wood doors that swung to behind us. I had the impression of being half underground, half submerged. I think I held my breath in anticipation of God-knows-what-horrors. We came to a door. Did it say Six Oaks? Were we accompanied? If so, I suppose it was our guide who knocked, for the door was locked. Someone unlocked and opened it and we stepped inside. The door was locked behind us. We gave our names again. It was not exactly bedlam. The room we had entered was large and wooden-floored like an old-fashioned schoolroom. I do not remember any particular noise. There was a man standing just inside the door, as if rooted to the floor, swaying slightly, looking blank and mumbling to himself. Probably I tried to smooth over the awkwardness, to speak to the nurses as if this were a perfectly usual and unexceptional sort of room to find oneself in, to introduce my son in a cordial, friendly manner, as if I were introducing him to a new school and new headmaster for the first time.

But Jeremy suddenly turned back. 'I'm not fucking staying here,' he said. He went to the door. I looked at the nurses. I remonstrated feebly. I understood entirely why he did not want to stay. The door was unlocked. 'Take me to King's Cross,' he said as soon as we were outside.

He wanted to go to Edinburgh, where he had been a student and still had some friends. Did I try to dissuade him? Did we talk on the way to the King's Cross station? I sympathised with him. I was still clutching at any straw that offered in those early days. Perhaps going back to Edinburgh, getting away from his family, finding himself once more in a place where he had been independent and happy, perhaps these things would cure him; perhaps he would find himself again. Or so I let myself hope, all too easily.

I left him at King's Cross. We said goodbye and I wished him luck. 'Let me know when you get there.'

Two or three days later I received a postcard. He sounded happy. Perhaps I had been right: perhaps just getting away was what he needed. A couple more days went by, then one afternoon about six o'clock my mother phoned. Jeremy had rung her from Newcastle, from a public telephone outside the railway station. He had no money, was very distraught and was talking nonsense,

Mum said. She had had nothing to hand to write with and had tried to memorise the number of the booth he had called from. By the time she had found a pencil the line had gone dead. She had rung the number as she remembered it but no one replied. She was afraid she had memorised it incorrectly. In the meantime she had spoken to the chief of police for Northumberland and explained that her grandson was penniless and unwell in the area of Newcastle station.

That was typical of my mother. I do not know how she did it. If I mentioned as a child that I might like to be a teacher, within a day or two she had spoken to the headmaster of Eton who told her that he would be very happy to speak to me. Or the Archbishop of Canterbury...

The Newcastle police chief told her that he would instruct his men to keep an eye out for Jeremy and that he should stay within the station precinct for as long as he could during the night and then catch the earliest train to London. Luckily he had a return ticket.

In spite of having the presence of mind to get in touch with the police chief, Mum was in a panic and so was I. I phoned the number she had given me. The phone rang and rang. I do not how long I waited, but a long time: far longer than normally one would wait for a phone that no one picked up. Miraculously, after somewhere between five and ten minutes, there was Jeremy's voice. 'It's me, Dad. Are you okay?' or some such completely redundant question. Obviously he was not okay. He was relieved to hear me. He said he had been collecting money in a pub nearby. He told me he had tried to climb the rocky face of Arthur's Seat in Edinburgh and fallen off and hurt his ankle. He had left Edinburgh by train, or so I thought, but why or when I could not make out, nor why he had got off in Newcastle. He said he had been out to the psychiatric hospital to interview patients, pretending he was a journalist. Just recently he has told me that he hitched to Newcastle with a doctor. Did the doctor take him to the hospital? He told me he had said he needed to be with schizophrenics. Did the hospital throw him out or threaten to take him in? I do not know.

Eventually we had to say goodbye. He promised to take the very first train in the morning. It left around six. I told him to stay in the station all night if he could and to go to the police if he needed help: to take a taxi when he got to London and I would pay.

Mum called two or three times, beside herself with worry. Her anxiety only made mine worse. She would never accept that there was nothing that could be done. 'Why don't you... What if you... Can't you get Professor what's-its phone number at two in the morning and get him out of bed and...?' 'Mum, what's the point? How can I? And what could he do anyway? He is only a doctor after all.' It was so easy to end up getting cross with her and shouting at her. I thought of perhaps driving to Newcastle through the night, but what if I could not find him? And what if he showed up here and I was gone?

I went to bed but could not sleep. In the small hours I heard terrible groans from Geoff's room and went to see what was going on. He was in agony from a horrible attack of piles. I drove him up to Accident and Emergency at the Royal Free Hospital. We checked him in and after a while I left. It was after four o'clock in the morning by then and I wanted to be within earshot of the phone. It was four hours before anyone came to see him, he told me later.

All morning I paced up and down, waiting to hear from Jeremy. Finally, about twelve, when I was beginning to wonder whether he had managed to get on the train, the phone rang. It was Jeremy. He was in a phone box in north London. He said he had spent the night, very frightened, on a bench outside the station. Then, having caught the train, he went up and down the carriages blessing people and saying *Ave Maria* and then, he said, he had hit a man in his compartment. Frightened at what he had done, he got off the train at Stevenage and boarded a later one. He kept seeing the man he had hit, he said, hovering around outside the phone box. I said, 'Don't worry. It can't be the same man. You've just given yourself a fright. He could not possibly know where you are. Get a taxi. Just stop a black cab and come here. Don't worry about the money. I'll pay when you get here.'

Two hours went by. I had no idea where he was. The phone rang and a girl's voice asked, 'Are you Jeremy's father? He's here. Can you come and get him? I'm frightened.'

He was in Holloway somewhere. I got straight in the car. It is hard to describe what you feel at such times. In a sense, nothing: just a blank, sick numbness. When I arrived and the door was opened to me, Jeremy was standing in the hall waiting. He was very still and very quiet. His face was blank and his eyes stared.

We got in the car. He had no luggage any more. It was difficult to work out exactly what had happened. I think it was probably later that he told me. He had gone down into an Underground station. There was a black man on the platform and he felt that this man was impelling him to jump under a train. So he left, leaving his Moroccan hold-all behind. Somewhere he had thrown his camera from a bridge. Then he had gone along a street putting coins on people's doorsteps. He had asked a black man if he could come in and watch TV.

He was frightened. He kept asking me to slow down – I was not going more than 20mph. 'Wait, wait, Dad!' he said. He did not want me to go near any red buses. I knew then what I had to do. The journey home would take us past the Royal Free. I did not say anything. When we got there, I simply turned into the Accident and Emergency bay. He did not protest. We went in together. Back again.

I do not remember how long we waited. Not very long, I think. Someone came and told me they were going to keep him in; they had a bed in one of the psychiatric wards, here, to my relief, in the Royal Free. On home ground. I can see it at the end of my street. I can be there in five minutes. Unlike the ghastly Friern. I went back to the hospital in the evening, with clean clothes, washing things and a couple of books. By that time Jeremy had tried to discharge himself and been 'sectioned.'

Thus, my son became a patient, acquired a psychiatric history. He still blames me sometimes for having brought this all about by taking him to the Royal Free that day. But schizophrenia is an illness, like cancer. It is not an existential matter. It is an illness, even if we do not yet understand its causes or its mechanisms, that damages the function of the brain in such a way that people's ability to reason normally, logically, to process and interpret the ordinary, humdrum experience of life in a normal, recognisable, intelligible way is fatally impaired: so that their view of how things are, of the experiences that they undergo, of the relationships they have with other people are not just bizarre, but incomprehensible to others not thus afflicted. Loss of reason: that is the distinguishing symptom. They go mad. They can hurt themselves, hurt others, die through believing that the only true diet for a human being is water and honey; set fire to their parents' or own homes, believing that only thus will the Pied Piper of Hamlin lead the angels back to Jerusalem; climb into the lions' den at the zoo to offer a nice Sainsbury's chicken to the poor hungry lion. Theirs is not some other but equal reality. They need treatment.

Chapter Three
Learning To Live With It

What do I remember of those years? Here and there a moment of hope, a moment of happiness, perhaps even a few days, maybe on occasion even a few weeks, of relative confidence. But overarching everything, anxiety: varying degrees of anxiety. Closely calibrated but chiefly in the upper register: from sustained worry – is he eating enough, what can I do to relieve the loneliness, to bring him some joy or fun, is he really suicidal? – to heart-in-mouth horror.

How many crises were there? How many times was he admitted to hospital? I do not remember.

That first hospital admission: thank God it took place at the Royal Free and not Friern. I do not think I could have managed Friern at that innocent stage of my career.

I would go up to the hospital nearly every afternoon, always with my heart in my mouth. I would try to bring something: cigarettes, some fruit, some clean clothes. His mum was good at that, buying him something clean and nice to wear. You are responsible for your own laundry on the psychiatric wards. Not surprisingly, people whose minds are distracted and tormented by madness do not often think about their appearance or their cleanliness. I guess if you were too filthy the nurses would do something about it. But scruffy and smelly: that is a regular part of the deal.

Psychiatric wards are frightening places when you are new to them. By you, I mean me, a visitor. God knows how fearful they must seem to someone condemned to stay in one. Jeremy was detained under the Mental Health Act. You can appeal to a tribunal and he did. Luckily, they rejected his appeal. He was in no state to return to ordinary life. So you do not know how long you are in for, for that is how it must feel: deprived of your liberty like a convict. And then there are the other people: aggressive, withdrawn, noisy, obsessive, frightened, shouting at Lord-knows-what, talking endlessly to themselves, strange in a thousand categories of strangeness, coming up to you with bizarre questions or requests. There is no escape from them.

Even in a modern hospital like the Royal Free, there was no privacy. Men and women slept separately but in the four-or-five-bed sleeping quarters a nylon curtain round the bed was all the privacy you enjoyed. People moaned, farted, played radios, lay all day in a stupor, smoked, called out, wandered. Some, thought to be seriously at risk of harming or killing themselves, had a permanent bodyguard, who watched over them day and night. They came from all kinds of background, many poor and homeless and uneducated.

Every visit to the hospital was an ordeal. I never knew how Jeremy would be. Indeed even today when, for the moment, things are as good as they have ever been, I am never sure what mood I will find him in. That uncertainty is terrible, wearing. To see your own child in this state, living in such conditions. For how long? For ever? He was drugged. He had to be. That is the only effective first line treatment for schizophrenia. He was batty, said odd things, things that did not connect. He would be angry with me. Sometimes he did not want to see me. Other times he asked me to get him out of there. He would make endless cups of tea and not drink them. That is a common symptom of mental illness. He smoked endlessly, dropping the ash on his bed, on the floor, in plates of congealed, half-eaten food that surrounded the bed. The sheets would be rucked up, dirty, the plastic anti-bed-wetting mattress exposed and he would lie on it, without ever taking his clothes off. I think he has probably spent most of the nights of the last twenty years in his clothes.

I fussed and bothered and twittered, trying to encourage him to clean up, use an ashtray, shave. You will feel better. Why not eat in the canteen with the others? You end up sounding critical all the time. In the end – a very long, long end – you train yourself to find fault, for that is how it must seem, less often. Ah, these lessons that have to be learnt.

And the unremitting hopelessness, the despair. Can anyone explain to you what schizophrenia is? What hope there is? This is what schizophrenia is: endless despair, endless, inconclusive treatment; endless clutching at little straws of betterness; endless realisation that that is all they are, is all there is.

He looked strained, lonely, frightened, pale. You want to know what is going on, what the prognosis is and no one can tell you. A nurse told me that parents are part of the trouble: a legacy of the teachings of RD Laing... That never happened again, I am glad to say. Some nurses were wonderful, kind, patient, reassuring, would even take the trouble to ring up at home sometimes if I were particularly worried.

There was nowhere to go at the Royal Free. You lived on neon-lit corridors. There was a sort of veranda area patients could use in good weather, gravelly, with a few wooden tables, but enclosed and scarcely natural, not at all uplifting.

I suppose I must have met Jeremy's consultant fairly early in this first admission. He was a neat, quiet, reserved man, and, as I was to learn over the years, kind, conscientious and understanding. I am sure I gave him a hard time to begin with, in my habitual aggressive manner, but then, I have also learnt, if you are not aggressive and pushy nothing happens.

I have had cause time and again to take up arms against what I can only call the system. Not the doctors, the medical staff – I have never had reason to quarrel seriously with them – but the bureaucratic system: the ill-defined and ill-co-ordinated network of arrangements for looking after mental patients outside hospital, for securing the social security benefits they need to live on, for finding them a place to live, for keeping an eye on them and recognising when they might be in a need of a new hospital admission and getting them admitted in time, before their condition worsens calamitously, for making sure that they take the medication which, more than anything else, keeps them out of hospital.

For all the professions of good intention, of commitment to enabling and empowering and returning to work and meaningful existence, social inclusion and all the rest of the brouhaha, my experience has been an object lesson in confusion, misunderstanding, lack of co-ordination, inability on the part of right hands to know what left hands are doing. For years the talk has been all about ending the revolving door syndrome – *i.e.* patients being endlessly discharged, then re-admitted to hospital after a relapse – and preventing patients from slipping through the net. Yet the net has always been – and in my opinion still is – so full of such big holes that even a whale could slip through without leaving a tear.

My memory of the detail of what happened in these early years is confused and unclear now. What happened in which hospital admission? Which crisis arose when, in relation to which other crisis?

That first hospital admission ended in discharge to a Richmond Fellowship residential home in Notting Hill. I think the admission lasted about six weeks. It is common for people to have to stay in hospital after they are considered well enough to leave simply because it is so difficult to find suitable accommodation. It is not easy to find a place in a Richmond Fellowship home or a *MIND* hostel or in any suitable kind of hostel, for there simply is not enough accommodation to go round.

Jeremy seemed to like the Richmond Fellowship to start with. It was a friendly unthreatening place, run along communal lines: the residents decided collectively how to organise their lives and share out chores and responsibilities. The house was attractive, a pretty Victorian semi on a quiet street. I took him there by car. It was like taking him to some new boarding school. I wanted to make his room homely for him, to make it as like home as possible, put up pictures and bookshelves. But he did not want that. He took just a few clothes. Besides, these places never are homely. They are hostels. People come and go. There is always that air of not-belonging-to-anyone. Others have slept in your bed before you and will do after you; others have pissed in your toilet and bathed in your bath. There are too many corridors and heavier-than-usual fire doors, too many pokey corners, because the building, designed as a family home, has been converted, divided up to provide bed-sits for strangers.

And you cannot stay there even if you want to, not beyond a couple of years: you are expected to move on. You are not allowed nowadays to become stuck in your ways, that is to say, to get used to a place and want to stay because it has become familiar, a home, in effect. That is to become institutionalised. You must be empowered, enabled: you must move on towards Recovery – but that is a story we shall come to later.

Jeremy was allocated a key worker, as is the custom in these places: that is, a person specifically designated as his minder/mentor/helper, who, in this instance, was a priest and former missionary. He was a nice, good man, who believed in what he called "hard love". I was not sure that was a sensible way of approaching schizophrenia, but he was a good man, concerned and ready to keep in touch with me and Jeremy's mother.

Jeremy took some courses, even acquired a certificate for some computer course. You start to think of things he might do, things that did not involve working too much with other people. He found other people difficult, was suspicious of them and often took against them for no obvious reason. That is paranoia and, sadly for him, has been one of the most disabling symptoms of his illness. I know other people, the children of friends, who have had a history quite as frequently punctuated by hospital admissions as Jeremy's and who have been in some ways crazier, but, untroubled by these paranoid feelings about others, have been just quietly dotty and much easier to deal with.

How many times have I thought of things he could do in order to give himself some kind of purpose, some kind of structure in his life: work in gardens, do voluntary work, some kind of computer work from home? But hearing voices, having strange, hostile feelings towards other people... all this wrecks your concentration and ability to keep to a routine.

It was not long before things started to go wrong again. There was an Italian girl he got a crush on. I do not know what happened. She said no and he slapped her? Something like that. He started refusing to go to the house collective meetings. One night he rang my doorbell at two in the morning. He was dressed only in pyjama trousers. He had come in a taxi. He was frightened, visibly frightened. He had been afraid he was going to jump out of the window of his room. I took him in and he lay on the sofa. He did not want to go bed, so I got some blankets and we spent the night on the sofas in my living room – scene of so many nights of misery and anxious talk! I tried to soothe him. He was physically sick, throwing up a thin bile. I did not know what to do. Might he really have jumped? Was he really suicidal? I mean, was there a real possibility that he might attempt suicide? People with schizophrenia do, around ten per cent, I believe. I know two people who have.

We spent the night with the light on. He has slept with the light on for years. He calmed down gradually and got a little sleep in the end. I did not. Geoff must have been sleeping upstairs. Jeremy got on well with him but could be jealous, jealous of anyone whom he might have to share my time with, to the point where often he would not stay with me if there were anyone else around.

One day I went to see him at the hostel. There was not much we could do. Usually he wanted to go for a walk and usually not much more than round the block and then he would want to go back to his room. Often he did not like meeting other people on the pavement and would make critical remarks about them, although they could not possibly have done anything to upset him. He had developed an odd habit of avoiding the cracks between paving stones, altering his stride so as not to step on the joins. And his own joints would crack, or so he said. 'Did you hear that?' he would say. His elbows, his knees, his wrists. The joint-cracking or crunching, as he sometimes calls it, continues to this day. I do not know whether it is pure delusion or some bizarre effect of the medication. He does not seem to worry about cracks in the pavement any more.

On this occasion he wanted to drive around. We got in the car. He was in a difficult and aggressive mood, I could see, although I had no idea why. Just the illness, probably, as Geoff would have said. But suddenly he reached across and grabbed me round the neck, pulling my head down over the gear lever and pummelling my head with his left fist. 'You *** scumbag,' he shouted at me, with other insults as well.

I freed myself with difficulty. We were just outside the hostel. I told him to get out of the car and left him. I was shocked but not badly hurt as he could not punch me effectively with his left hand. There are no reasons for such behaviour. I have long since given up seeking explanations. He always says sorry within a day or two.

On another occasion the phone rang and he asked me in a frightened voice to come round and take him to hospital: he was not feeling well. (For years I have hated telephone calls, especially early in the morning or late at night. So often they have boded ill.) We went straight to Accident and Emergency at St Charles Hospital. It must have been about ten in the evening. We waited and waited. We were seen around two in the morning. To my surprise Jeremy stayed with me. Normally he is very impatient and if what he wants does not happen quickly he is off. The staff were perfectly nice, just busy and short-handed. Always you are asked the same questions when schizophrenia is mentioned. Do you hear voices? What do they say to you? Is there any history of schizophrenia in the family?

When is an emergency an emergency, one wonders? He was not admitted. Probably there were not any beds. As he seemed less agitated we went back to the hostel.

*

I could not eat. I could not sleep. I had a permanent hollow ache of anxiety in the pit of my stomach. I talked to Geoff. I talked to a woman friend, recently widowed; she too had a son suffering from schizophrenia. One evening I went to dinner at a neighbour's. It must have been during Jeremy's first admission. We ate in a bay window and it was light. It must have been summer. The question of schizophrenia came up. I must have mentioned it. I tried not to talk about it all the time, especially with people who did not know me. One of the other guests, a woman, said immediately, 'Do you know about the National Schizophrenia Fellowship?' I did not. 'It's an organisation started by people like you, parents with children suffering from schizophrenia. They have lots of local support groups. I have got the phone number at home. I'll give it to you.'

She did and I made contact with the nearest group. It was big and flourishing, run by a couple whose own son, like mine, had fallen ill shortly after finishing university. They met twice a month, once in Golders Green and once at a local hospital. The first meeting was, you might say, more social; it was better attended and speakers were invited. The second was more like a workshop, an opportunity to discuss individuals' particular problems and consider practical ways of dealing with them. There was always at least one professional present at these latter meetings, a community psychiatric worker, kind and sympathetic, who has been with us throughout the twenty years I have been involved: a rare example of continuity and commitment in a world where staff turnover is even more frequent than in teaching.

There were fifteen or twenty people present at the first meeting I went to. I was the only newcomer. When the business of the day had been attended to, Jenni – alas, now dead – who ran the more social side of things, turned to me and asked me to tell my story. And at once I knew I was among friends. Here there was no need to explain the most bizarre of events, the craziest of utterings, the fear, anxiety and frustration involved in dealing with this whackiest of illnesses. There was nothing I could tell the others that they had not experienced for themselves and many had survived experiences far more horrific than any I have ever had to cope with – and there is a strange comfort in that: knowing that your lot is not as bad as it could be. Finding myself among these people I felt an unimaginable sense of relief and comfort.

For the first time since Jeremy began to act so strangely I felt at home and not alone: and have continued for twenty years to draw comfort from finding myself in their company. Our numbers have dwindled severely, for various reasons, but the few regulars are all familiar faces, all been at it much longer than me.

Whether the comfort had anything to do with the fact that so many of those who attended our group were Jewish, I do not know. I suspect yes. There was a warmth and intimacy and lack of barriers that is very un-English. Jenni and Tony, her husband, who still marshals us at the age of ninety, were themselves a wonderful combination of personalities: she, the epitome of the all-embracing mother, able to make even the most unlovely feel loved; he, the clear-thinking, analytical, political campaigner.

Several of the group had German, Austrian and other central European backgrounds. They were tough and humorous – and, God, is that important when you live with such awfulness – able to make fun of themselves and light of the awful situations they lived with: one, in particular, herself a retired psychiatrist. I always remember her describing a visit of the so-called Crisis Intervention Team, summoned to assess her son. When the doorbell rang he went to let them in and ushered them into the living room, explaining that he was terribly worried about his parents; he thought they were not well at all. And away went the Team, reporting there was nothing much wrong with the son. He would say to his mother: 'I don't know why you keep insisting you are my mother. If you would stop that, I could think of you as quite a nice old lady.' In the end he became obsessed with the notion that honey and water was all he required as a diet. He had no contact with the social services and would not see his mother. Eventually, seeing no light in his flat for several days, she broke in and found him unconscious, almost dead. He has been confined to a wheelchair in a nursing home ever since.

The majority of people who attend our group have always been women, mothers mostly, for obvious reasons. There were a few "sufferers", as they are called. It is a horrible word – not as bad as service-user or, worse, user, which is the current jargon – but none of us likes to say "schizophrenics". Calling our offspring that seems insulting: it is too much like saying loonies or maniacs or madmen or else it seems too clinical, like referring to people with cancer as the cancerous, as if that were the defining aspect of their identity.

Some of these women are truly heroic. Rather than leave their sick sons or daughters to the tender mercies of an impersonal system of care that is unable to provide decently for them they have dedicated their lives to looking after them at home. Some do it with extreme fortitude. Others have clearly destroyed their own lives in making this sacrifice. I remember in particular a woman who had dedicated herself to the care of both a husband and a son: she seemed utterly exhausted, pale and ghostlike.

There are cultural differences too. I think of a Greek woman and an English woman married to a Greek. Both had great difficulty in getting their husbands to accept that their sons – that of course makes it more unbearable for the fathers – were ill and not merely wilful good-for-nothings. These attitudes are not confined to the eastern Mediterranean.

It was towards the end of this first year of diagnosed illness – my *annus horribilis* – that I met one of my first cousins for the first time. She had come from New Zealand. She was the daughter of my mother's brother. He had had a very chequered career, never seeming to keep any job for very long, often being out of work and in effect drifting. I had heard my mother speak of him as feckless and irresponsible. She and her sister had paid for him to return to England and looked after him on various occasions. He would get a job teaching biology in Nigeria and before the first term was out there would be trouble: back he would come, expecting his sisters to bail him out.

I told my cousin of my troubles with my son. 'My brother is schizophrenic,' she said at once. 'He has been ill for years. He goes off and disappears, living rough, and no one knows where he is for months at a time.' I told her that the doctors always asked me if there were any history of schizophrenia in the family – there often is – and I said no, not as far as I know. 'Oh,' she said, 'Dad has been diagnosed as well.'

I rang my mother and told her what my cousin, her niece, had said, that both her brother and her nephew had diagnoses of schizophrenia and that this had been confirmed by her sister-in-law, whom I had also just met for the first time. 'Nonsense,' said my mother. 'Besides I wouldn't listen to anything that woman says.' "That woman", my uncle's first wife, had never been approved of in the family. I said, 'Well, it is hardly something she would make up, at least not where her own son is concerned.'

A couple of days later I found a message on my answer machine from my mother's sister, "the bossy one". I did not reply, knowing what it would be about. So she wrote me a letter, saying it was nonsense to claim that her brother suffered from schizophrenia. When he was young they had taken him to see Sir Somebody Something, the famous psychiatrist and friend of her father-in-law, himself the famous brain surgeon, Sir Somebody Something Else. 'There is nothing wrong with young G,' they ruled. 'He was merely immature and feckless.'

People do not like to own up to mental illness in the family. The reasons may be understandable, but denying it does not help anyone. Awareness of the history partly explains an otherwise apparently inexplicable change in a loved one and may also be a useful warning: there is no inevitability in the legacy of schizophrenia from one generation to the next, but there is no doubt that the risk is there.

*

Just looking back over the history of this illness is horribly painful. I just do not want to recall the details. Deteriorating memory partly alleviates the pain, but I am also aware that my mind is putting up an obstinate resistance to being made to live it all again.

There were a couple of hospital admissions during my son's stay with the Richmond Fellowship. One, I think, was at the Royal Free and one at Friern. I always preferred the Royal Free, as I can be there in five minutes and the ward staff were always willing to let me in even outside formal visiting hours. Visitors are not two a penny on psychiatric wards; there is no danger of overcrowding, at least not by visitors.

Visits are always distressing but you sort of get used to it. Entrance used to be through the ward for anorexics: poor emaciated things, but at least they were more or less in their right minds. It is the helplessness and hopelessness of psychiatric patients that distressed me most and the sense that your own child had really fallen to the very bottom of the heap of humanity, where he had to rub shoulders in the most intimate ways with the most uncouth, ill-mannered, ignorant, uneducated and, to me at least, alien elements of society: an awful and distressing equality in madness.

Then, sometimes, I think that in some peculiar way the illness actually protects those who suffer from it from the realisation of quite how devastating it is and quite how terrible their plight. At least I hope that is so and I try to take some comfort from that. It certainly does seem to protect my son from any other kind of illness, even the common cold, though I fear the long-term consequences of his heavy smoking.

It is so hard to know. The thought that your child's entire life is unadulterated hell is hard to bear. There does seem to be some happiness – interludes, at least: coffee in the sunshine, a pretty student nurse, no matter how unattainable. And there are adventures: an affair with a young Portuguese girl, a fellow patient. She had one of the few single bedrooms. I never quite understood on what basis they were allocated to patients; maybe everyone got a turn. But on this occasion it certainly facilitated the affair. The pair were caught in bed together. There was a terrible to-do because it was thought the girl was under sixteen, although that turned out not to be the case.

On another occasion there was a pale Irish girl who wore a great mouthful of crimson lipstick like a gash. That time we discovered that Jeremy had actually been down to the Town Hall to publish the banns, which just shows that some human instincts are too strong even for paranoia, agoraphobia and terrifying delusion.

Friern I dreaded because it was so fearful of aspect and it took me half an hour and more to drive there. As I tried to go almost every day, that added up to many hours in the week. But perhaps it offered a calmer and safer environment for patients. There was much more space, both within the building and without.

We arrived on the scene, became the familiars of the world of madness, at the very end of the ascendancy of the bins, when they had already been consigned to the category of unmentionably cruel and shameful human behaviour, like slavery and the workhouse. But I have talked to people who remember the old bins, who say that their therapeutic effectiveness is much traduced by the current cliché view of them as harsh prisons in which society's weakest and most ill-adapted were heartlessly dumped: out of sight, out of mind. They were on the contrary havens of peace and security, with farms, gardens and workshops in which their patients could find some fulfilling occupation...

Just mentioning the name of Friern brings back the memory of that drive. I even feel again the tensing in my entrails, the sick anxiety, and I can see in my mind's eye, almost feel the jolts and turns of the roads that lead to it. Once there, once I had seen Jeremy, I felt better: at least the tension eased, even when he was not well, as if his continued physical existence were by itself reassuring. I still feel that apprehension every time I go to visit him in hospital, in fact even when I go to visit him at home, still, after twenty years: what state is he going to be in?

My wife today, whom I did not even know in those days, who is in every way supportive, my very present help in trouble, feels, I think, that I fuss and worry more than necessary. But she has never had children herself and herein lies, I think, the crucial difference. A parent, equipped by nature, has a built-in alarm system that is permanently active, albeit, perhaps for most, in sleep mode once the children have grown up. My alarm system has had cause to shrill so often that sleep mode has vanished from its repertoire. Schizophrenia is not in itself a life-threatening illness, as a Greek psychiatrist friend pointed out to me long ago: but it does so affect the mood and behaviour of the person suffering from it that you never know what you are going to find and you can never forget that it can provoke behaviour that could be life-threatening. The great comfort of support groups is that everybody there knows this: they too are on permanent alert, listening for signs that may presage trouble, emergency. What is tedious and repetitive for others is just part of everyday experience for them.

Usually, at Friern, we walked in the grounds, even if it was raining. It gave us something to do. It was too depressing sitting in the cafeteria, which must once have been the hospital refectory, drinking tea out of polystyrene cups at tables from which previous occupants' slops had not been wiped, mostly in silence, while Jeremy sucked at a succession of roll-ups. Sometimes, a "friend" would come up and say hello or even join us. I put "friend" in inverted commas because for all his many hospital admissions where often the same faces show up time and again he has not made or maintained more than one or two friendships. That has always seemed strange to me; I would have thought that there could be comfort in having a few friends with whom you share this ghastly experience. I do not know whether it is simply Jeremy's own temperament that accounts for this or whether there is something in the illness that makes friendship a difficult thing to achieve, a preoccupation with things, with events going on inside you that cannot be communicated, that looks like an extreme form of self-obsession. Isolation and friendlessness are certainly among the most frequent, and saddest, concomitants – I am tempted to say symptoms, even – of the illness. There is also a peculiar kind of democracy about the illness, as if it made all distinctions of education, upbringing or class almost completely irrelevant. It is almost impossible to tell on a psychiatric ward where people come from in society, apart from undisguisable distinctions like race. Perhaps not making friends on wards is a way of protecting yourself, of guarding a little bit of your "real" identity, of preserving a core of your old pre-illness self, of your "proper" life. I do not want to live with a lot of nutters, he says, when I suggest that sheltered accommodation might be the safest way to live. He often refers to events and people from pre-illness times, when his life too looked as if it would follow the expected and normal course.... Caroline, Paul, Bethan... So hard. Your friends all turn away from you. You have dropped off the planet as far as they are concerned. They have their lives, their wives, their careers... There is no place for a lunatic. One man has kept in touch faithfully, by letter and email. He has been abroad most of these long years, which perhaps has made it easier, but he has kept in touch. God bless him.

So, I think we both preferred to walk during visits, two or three times round the huge rambling complex of buildings, redeveloped now as flats (did any of the money from the sale of this huge site find its way back into caring for its former patients?). In front there were ill-kept lawns scattered with trees. At the back were the ruins of kitchen gardens, with apple and pear trees and raspberry cages that had once been worked by patients from the hospital. Once we heard music coming from what looked like a long-abandoned potting shed. There was a hole in the fence enclosing the gardens and I went through to investigate. Everything looked neat and ship-shape, clearly the work of a human hand. And the music was coming unmistakably from the open door. I put my head round it and there was a man sitting at a table. He looked pretty surprised. The interior was well swept, the man's coat hung from a hook, a broom was propped against the wall. It must have been in 1991 or '92, at the latest. The man said he was the gardener; he had been coming and spending every day in this shed since 1984, when the gardens had last been cultivated!

Friern was also the scene of the most frightening visit I have ever paid to my son. It was summer;.I had just returned from a trip to France and Jeremy had been admitted in my absence. I went into the ward and could not see him. A nurse directed me to a little courtyard outside, enclosed by a high metal fence topped with revolving sections of razor wire. Jeremy lay on a bench, white as a sheet, with his knees drawn up to his chest, not in a posture of relaxation but of extreme tension. His eyes were blank and staring. All humanity seemed to have drained from him; he looked like a poor mad thing. I thought I was going to die. My child, my child. Mad. This time I have lost him. He will never be human again.

It was the medication, the nurse told me. He had had to be sedated. It would wear off.

You have to trust the doctors and by and large I do; I have never had occasion seriously to question the treatment they were prescribing. There may be some who resort to heavy doses of medication more readily than others. It is difficult to eradicate all thoughts of *One Flew over the Cuckoo's Nest* from one's mind. But they have to deal with difficult, even dangerous situations: if someone goes berserk, as my son himself admits that he has done, they have to do something to protect the lives of staff, other patients, the berserk one himself. Jeremy says that once three or four hefty male nurses floored him because he knocked over a bookcase. That seems rather extreme, but who knows... I was not there.

One of the things you come to realise very quickly when confronted with this horrible illness is that the doctors – the scientists – do not actually know very much about it or have many weapons in their armoury for dealing with it. Full of foolish and anguished hope you ask what the prognosis is, what the likely outcomes may be, and in truth no answer is forthcoming. People recover from breakdowns, whatever they are: perhaps they are just the reactions of people overwhelmed by events in their lives, not really illnesses. But recovery from schizophrenia or madness? Some people seem to get off more lightly than others. A few manage to hold jobs of one kind or another some of the time, even maintain relationships like marriage. For some their symptoms seem less acute than for others; they have fewer hospital admissions. I have come to think that this is as much a function of someone's personality and temperament as anything else: you can be dotty and docile – much easier to deal with – or dotty and aggressive. In my son's case I often think that what makes him difficult is his very independence of spirit, his determination not to give in, not to be defined by his illness: a kind of crazy courage, which I cannot but admire and in some perverse way also support, although it also incidentally causes me much pain and difficulty.

There is no prognosis, there is no charted course of recovery; no one can say, follow this treatment and little by little the illness will clear up. Coming to terms with this, this certainty of a future full of perpetual anxiety, full of perpetual uncertainty, this absolute lack of hope, is very very hard. So hard, in fact, that you never really accept it: always you deceive yourself with little glimmers of hope... and rumours of hope. So and so's son or daughter has been really well on a diet of eggs and carrots; so and so has switched to a new medication and it has completely transformed his life... Momentarily your hopes are raised. Perhaps there really is a miracle medicine, if only I can get my son on it. If I could get him to go for a second opinion at the Maudsley, which is the great centre for research in psychiatric medicine in this country. They have close links with the National Schizophrenia Fellowship and will give any of us a really sympathetic hearing. But my son will not go. Even when I explain to him that Clozapine, for this is the miracle medicine that we keep hearing is the only truly effective anti-psychotic drug, could make him feel so much better, he does not want to hear about it. It requires regular blood tests, for ever, because it can cause damage in a few people to their white blood cell count.

And then you meet people who say, well, my son was on Clozapine and it did not appear to do him any good. Then you feel jealous of those whose children – they can be sixty – seem to be doing so well. Then you hear that so and so, who had even managed to hold quite a sophisticated job, has killed himself. Or x is setting fire to her parents' home again. Just yesterday a friend told me that his former brother-in-law who for years had worked as a rent officer and then librarian had recently, aged nearly sixty, attacked and wrecked his sister's house. And you think, oh well, at least, things are not as bad as that; they could be worse. You can feel sorry for someone else and derive a little bit of satisfaction from that.

You feel there should be a treatment. Is not that after all what medicine is about? Is not that why my son has been taken into hospital, so he can be treated and made better? When you begin to realise that there is no better, merely an alleviating of the acuteness of the symptoms, a lessening of the craziness, a return to just the normal state of dottiness, for that essentially is all the medication can achieve, you are filled with despair and with frustration against the doctors. But they are not to blame, for that at least: not enough research has been done; we simply do not know enough about what causes the kind of damage in the brain that can so affect a person's mind.

If I had one reproach against the doctors, it was against their aloofness, the impression they gave of not being interested in what happened to their patients once they had left hospital, as if in a way it was no business of theirs. Theirs was the domain of science; it was their job to prescribe and oversee the administration of medication – though it was never very clear what criteria determined their choices other than habit or personal preference. Beyond the walls of the hospital where the messy business of life took place was a territory which did not concern them.

I can think of two extenuating circumstances that partly excuse this attitude. On the one hand, there were the old hierarchical values of the profession: the consultant as God, attended by a bevy of subservient acolytes who trembled at his displeasure and quivered with eagerness to implement his commands. (I once worked in the catering department of St Thomas's Hospital, paying the food bills, and saw with my own eyes how the surgeons dined on grouse and cognac while the *hoi polloi* got bangers and mash!) And, on the other hand, Care in the Community was still in its infancy: confining the mentally ill to life in the long-stay bins had been abandoned in favour of the more humane policy of looking after them in the community. But no one had really foreseen the likely problems that that would entail or made provision for the resources in money, staff, bricks and mortar necessary to make it work, let alone worked out how the various bodies and bureaucracies charged with providing the different aspects of this care were going to divide their responsibilities and co-ordinate their activities.

You take a person suffering from a psychotic illness into hospital, control his symptoms with medication and then discharge him into the community. Where is he going to live? Who is going to keep an eye on him? Who is going to make sure he has enough money to live on and spends it sensibly, that he does not spend it all on drink and not have enough left over to keep warm? Who is going to see that he has a reasonable diet? Who is going to make sure he takes the medication without which he will go round the bend again? What are they going to do about it if he refuses to take his medication – which is itself one of the classic symptoms of schizophrenia? Are they going to compel him? Does the law allow them to? Who is going to help him keep himself and his home clean? If you go around looking like a tramp and smelling, you are not likely to make a lot of friends or make it easy for yourself to conduct even ordinary everyday transactions like buying things in shops. When you get on the bus people move away from you. If you can get on a bus, if your illness does not make you so paranoid about other people that you are not too frightened by such an experience... Who is going to call the plumber when the sink gets immovably blocked by accumulated muck from unwashed dirty plates or a cleaner when strange cultures grow in your glasses?

And what sort of accommodation are people going to live in? Their own flats? How are they going to find them, when even the simplest of tasks and bureaucratic procedures are too much for their ruined concentration and damaged minds? Does the Council hold a reserve of suitable flats for such vulnerable people, secure from the teasing attentions of feral teenagers and not too exposed to neighbours and their noise, which might inspire troublesome paranoid thoughts? Of course not: it has sold them all off and its estates have become the resort of the defeated lumpenproletariat and the unassimilated poor of many nations and creeds: hardly a haven for those in need of security and calm.

Sheltered accommodation, as it is euphemistically called? Hostels? I have yet to see one I would want to live in. They feel even more institutional than hospital wards to me. Your fellows can include people with a history of homelessness and drinking, people of all ages. There is a community, but false because forced and not wished for. Kitchens, sitting-rooms, bathrooms are shared. The only privacy is your bedroom. Your neighbours may be even crazier than yourself. The building is probably converted, not purpose-built, its interior spaces poky; there is nothing private or personal or homely about it at all.

And then there is bed and breakfast...

When Jeremy was first ill, patients discharged from hospital became the charges of the Social Services – if they were officially homeless. Things are not a lot better now, but in those days there was very little cooperation between the hospital and the social services, between the social services and the patient's parents or informal carers. Nobody informed anybody of what they were doing or even trying to do. You could not even discover what provisions, if any, had been made for the care of your child: what would happen in a crisis, how was a crisis to be recognised, who was responsible for knowing, for acting?

In the course of one of these early admissions to Friern hospital – October 1991 – it was made clear that my son could not return to the Richmond Fellowship. I think the pretext was that he had used up his time there and it was their policy to "move people on". Contrary to their assurances to me, they let him go without making any attempt to find him further suitable accommodation. As the time approached for his discharge from Friern there was nowhere for him to go. Camden's social workers were on strike, indeed had been for a whole year. I did not know who to turn to. Apparently no one was prepared to take the responsibility of finding him somewhere to live.

And then I discovered that there was one woman social worker who as a matter of principle had refused to join the strike, Jill Gipps. I forget how I found her but I remember speaking to her on the phone at Friern and she invited me to come and meet her. It was a grim wet day, an appropriate reflection of my mood. Especially in those early days I was tormented by the vision of my son ending up on the streets a down-and-out. It is the fate of many. I spent a week at Crisis at Christmas once, where I noticed significant numbers of people suffering from schizophrenia. When Jill Gipps promised she would not let my son be discharged without a home to go to, I could not restrain my tears. She said the best thing was to get him registered as a vulnerable Homeless Person so that the Council would then have a responsibility to house him. His application was made on March 10th 1992 when Jill Gipps was given to understand that he could be housed at a St Mungo's hostel close to me in a matter of weeks. He came to live with me in the meantime but his condition began to deteriorate and he was admitted to Friern once again in May.

What had happened to the promise of a place at St Mungo's? The Homeless Persons Department had lost his application and did not find it again for eight weeks. He was finally registered as a homeless person on May 25th, by which time he was in hospital again and St Mungo's no longer had any vacant places. There followed a prolonged stay in hospital while he waited for a vacancy to occur – not the last prolonged period of hospitalisation occasioned by housing problems rather than illness.

Of all the many professional people who have played a role in our lives during the last twenty years – most of them scarcely more than walk-on parts, Jill Gipps stands out as the only one who has taken an initiative she did not have to take. The only one who came to me, as it were, rather than re-acted to pressure from me.

I was lucky enough also at this time to have a generous Greek mother-in-law, who gave me enough money to buy a flat for my son. Jill Gipps contacted the Council and discovered that they would be prepared to pay Housing Benefit to me as my son's landlord. I could not have afforded to run the flat without receiving some income from it. 'It seems to me,' she wrote, 'that the situation where Jeremy became your tenant would be the most advantageous to all parties,' and she wished me luck with the flat-hunting.

There have been plenty of people who have thought that Jeremy was not well enough to live on his own and there have certainly been problems over the years and a lot of anxiety and extra work for me. But I would like to record the fact that of all the professional people I have had dealings with because of Jeremy's illness Jill Gipps alone offered warm, unequivocal words of encouragement and advice, trusting in her own humanity and experience, unafraid of possible comebacks, unconcerned with all the provisos and hedging that the cautious bureaucratic mind is heir to. And as for my former mother-in-law, I dread to think where we might all have ended up without her generosity.

Chapter Four
Care Plan

By coincidence the St Mungo's hostel where Jeremy eventually found a place was in the next street to the cousin who had just arrived from New Zealand, whom I had never met before, and from whom I heard for the first time that there was a history of schizophrenia in our family, in both her brother and her father, my uncle.

It was a pretty street lined with cherry trees, in a respectable part of town, safe, close to me, close to Jeremy's mother, close to the hospital, close to the Tube, though I should not think he has ventured down there more than half a dozen times in twenty years. There was a large garden at the back that I tried to encourage him to get involved with, believing that growing things, manual work, working with nature would by itself have some therapeutic value. Perhaps it does. I believe it does, but I have never been able to persuade him to try this kind of thing. He is a city boy, unlike me. Perhaps I should have brought my children up in the country... and thus the guilt begins to work: I let my children down, I did not even baptise them, I made them live in the city, I left them when they were too young, I did not give them half the things my parents gave me...

As hostels go, it was a nice one, but it was a hostel. Corridors and fire doors and gloomy unclaimed places, where at any moment you might meet another furtive creature trying to get to his room without being seen, without having to meet anyone else.

Jeremy had a key worker. There were staff present during the daytime. The key worker was his designated member of staff. I do not know what training they received. Mostly they have always seemed to me kind, genuine people, eager to help – no one else would undertake such a thankless, poorly paid task. But Jeremy does not like hostels and rarely is prepared to co-operate with any such "helpers", whether social workers, community psychiatric workers or key workers. It was not long before there were problems; he was accused of being aggressive and uncooperative.

While he was in hospital, it was upsetting contemplating his future and wondering what would happen to him, but at least I felt safe, in the knowledge that he was safe, even if unhappy. It should have been like this when he was in a hostel, but it never was because he so disliked it he soon fell foul of the regime and then there arose again the threat of eviction and further uncertainty.

*

Around this time my local National Schizophrenia Fellowship group co-ordinator asked if I would like to join the steering committee for the organisation's London and south-east England branch. I am not a committee man. I am impatient with minutes and resolutions. I understand nothing about accounts. But they needed people, Tony said, with direct experience of the illness and who were not afraid to speak out.

So I joined and dutifully went to the meetings. It gave me the feeling that I was doing something, something to help my son and others like him. I do not think I made any great contribution, because so much of the business was business: money matters, the funding of projects, the appointment of staff. Already the organisation had begun to change from being a vehicle for campaigning on behalf of people with schizophrenia to becoming itself a provider of services. Obviously it could not compete with the NHS: we persuaded ourselves that we were pointing the way (leading excellence is how they put it now), setting up housing projects, advisory services, support for carers, employment projects. Setting an example to the government of what sort of thing should be done and how. Critics among the founder members of the NSF accused us of turning it into NSF plc – a criticism which events have shown to be correct and one which anticipated a transformation that in my view has not helped any of us. It was a pardonable mistake for it came about because the

Care-in-the-Community revolution had not been properly prepared and the public health services were simply not providing the necessary care.

At least I met some good and generous people, people who gave their time and money to the cause of the mentally ill, not all of them even with a personal stake. For me just that sense of being part of a group with a common and urgent purpose was a help, a kind of therapy, illusory though the sense of anything achieved may have been.

Fired up with campaigning zeal I went on a Kilroy Silk television programme and made some noisy intervention against a Tory MP. I phoned in to one or two radio programmes. I started going to Carers' groups. I remember an old lady saying to me, 'It's all right for you educated ones.' Well, it was not all right: I suffered too, but I assumed she meant that at least I could speak out in public.

I did feel – and still do – that those of us who are not afraid to stand up in public and are articulate enough to overcome the pressures of personality should do so. We have a duty to speak on behalf of our comrades in pain. We know where it hurts. The professionals in the social services, local government and charity bureaucracies do not and, worse, being the creatures of passing fads they are often blinded to the truth by both their own ideological training and their understandable desire for career advancement.

I had begun to feel by this time that there was a real possibility that the nightmare of my son living on the streets could become reality. The arrangements for looking after him outside hospital seemed so loose and haphazard. Who had ultimate responsibility for decisions about what should happen to him? What was supposed to happen and when, if he suffered a relapse? Who was responsible for identifying the relapse? Who was going to decide that his health had deteriorated enough and the time had come to admit him to hospital? Could we be sure that there would always be a hospital bed when he needed it and preferably at the Royal Free?

I had learnt through my association with the NSF that there was supposed to be something called a Care Programme

Approach which entailed holding multi-disciplinary meetings before a patient was discharged from hospital at which representatives of the various agencies responsible for looking after him – medical, social, housing – would agree on a "care package". One individual would be named as the person charged with seeing that all these recommendations were actually put into practice. The arrangements were supposed to provide a "seamless network of care" so that patients would not "fall through the net" and be caught up in the "revolving door syndrome", as the ghastly jargon has it.

What is a Care Plan?

I was sent a Department of Health document called an *Annex: The Care Programme Approach for People with a Mental Illness Referred to the Specialist Psychiatric Services*. Its origins apparently lay in a 1975 White Paper. The section entitled *Implementation* says that 'it is for health authorities, in discussion with consultant psychiatrists, nurses, social workers and other professional staff, and social services authorities to seek to establish suitable local arrangements, and to see that they are maintained in the context of purchaser/provider arrangements post-1 April 1991.' It goes on to say that among specific issues that all authorities will need to address are: inter-professional working; involving patients and carers; and keeping in touch with patients and ensuring agreed services are provided.

Under the heading *Inter-professional working* it states that 'modern psychiatric practice calls for effective inter-professional collaboration... and proper consultation with patients and carers.'

Under *Involving Carers* we are told: 'Relatives and other carers often know a great deal about the patient's earlier life (*sic*), previous interests, abilities and contacts and may have personal experience of the course of his/her illness spanning many years... Carers often make a major and valued contribution to the support received by many people with a mental illness being treated in the community. Where a care programme depends on such a contribution it should be agreed in advance with the carer who should be properly advised both about such aspects of the patient's condition as is necessary for the support to be given and how to secure professional advice and support, both in emergencies and on a day-to-day basis...'

Further: 'Sometimes patients being treated in the community will decline to co-operate with the agreed care programmes. An informal patient is free to discharge himself from patient status at any time, but often treatment may be missed due to the effects of the illness itself and with limited understanding of the likely consequence...

'Every reasonable effort should be made to maintain contact with the patient and, where appropriate, his/her carers, to find out what is happening, to seek to maintain the therapeutic relationship and, if this is not possible, to try to ensure that the patient and carer knows how to make contact with his key worker or other professional staff... It is particularly important that the patient's general practitioner is kept fully informed of a patient's situation and especially of his or her withdrawal... from a care programme...'

All these recommendations supposed, by 1991, to be guiding practice in the care of people like my son. Yet I had not come across anything like this at this point. I started to agitate.

In the pages that follow I have quoted from the voluminous correspondence I saved from my exchanges with various agencies in my attempts to find out at that time what my son's Care Plan or Programme was supposed to be. The lack of urgency, the lack of co-ordination, the sheer muddle and contradiction, in effect, the total absence of a system at all is embarrassingly and alarmingly obvious.

What is the Care Plan for my son: letters to the consultant
On November 18th 1991 I wrote to my son's consultant, asking for an appointment to discuss my son's situation. I pointed out that I had already written once, three weeks previously, and received no reply and that, in addition, I had made the same request to his secretary three times on the phone since August, again without receiving a reply.

By the end of January, I had still not received a reply. Six months had elapsed since my first attempt to arrange a meeting.
On January 26th 1992 I wrote again, enclosing copies of my previous letter:

'This is now my third written attempt to elicit some response from you...

'I should appreciate a reply to this letter at your earliest convenience. I am going on the *Kilroy* television programme tomorrow, when the topic under discussion is mental illness. I hope I shall be able to make some of these points. Since joining the National Schizophrenia Fellowship I find my experience with the Health Service is pretty universal where mental illness is concerned.

'If I don't get a reply from you, I shall send copies of the correspondence to my MP and the NSF.

'If it turns out that some misunderstanding accounts for the fact that I have not heard from you before, please excuse my belligerence. I am sure you can appreciate that being left in the dark is very distressing for parents in our situation.'

On January 30th I at last received a reply: 'I am sorry you have had difficulty in getting through to me... phone my office... so that an early appointment can be made.'

We met, I suppose. I have no recollection of the meeting. I came to like the man. He was kind, honourable and decent. His special interest was, I think, eating disorders, but I never had the slightest reason to doubt his competence or the correctness of his treatment of my son. It was just that he was completely unused to having to deal with the public or this ill-rehearsed system of looking after the mentally ill in the so-called community.

On May 26th 1993, Jeremy fell ill again or, rather, relapsed again and was re-admitted, this time to the Royal Free. Earlier that same day it had been clear that things were not going at all well. He had been to see his GP, a local doctor, who said he was suffering from 'flu symptoms and told him to take two paracetamol. He then came round to see me. He was talking about going to Libya to speak to Col. Gaddafi, which, even without any medical knowledge, I thought was a somewhat unusual 'flu symptom. Suddenly he became very angry – probably because I was trying to talk him into going into hospital – and cracked me on the jaw with a straight right, splitting my lip. He calmed down very quickly, was terribly contrite and agreed it would be a good thing if he were to go into hospital for a while. I called the consultant who told us we could come up to the ward and he would make sure everything was ready for Jeremy to be admitted. We walked up to the Royal Free together. It was a relief to be going there and not to Friern. We were done with Friern at last; I have never been there again.

Jeremy was admitted as a voluntary patient. A few weeks later he was discharged and returned to St Mungo's, still without a Care Plan.

On July 9th 1993, I wrote to the consultant:
'First, let me thank you for the interest you have taken in my son. Secondly, may I assure you that the list of people to whom I am sending copies of this correspondence is in no way intended as a slight to you personally nor as an indication of any doubt on my part as to your competence. It is just that, now that Jeremy has been admitted to hospital five times since 1990, I would like to clarify once and for all precisely what continuing provision of care for him, his mother and I can assume the "system" is making. And since you are the senior consultant I do not know who else to turn to.

'I was under the impression that patients discharged from psychiatric wards were to be provided with a Care Plan setting out what continuing treatment was envisaged for them and naming at least one individual who would be responsible for keeping an eye on them. Does such a Plan exist for Jeremy? Do you know where I can get a copy of it?

'The most frustrating thing for us as parents and carers, apart from the intractable nature of the illness, is the lack of information and communication between the various agencies involved in Jeremy's case. I know, for instance, that the staff at the St Mungo's hostel where he lives have been very concerned about the lack of communication with the Royal Free. Most importantly, they have never – in nearly a year now – been informed about the level of his medication. And apparently his GP actually refused to communicate this information to them prior to Jeremy's most recent admission to the Royal Free on May 26th on the grounds that it would damage his relationship with Jeremy. Furthermore, Jeremy gave me to understand at the time of his relapse that his medication had been, or was about to be, reduced. Is that true? Could that have had anything to do with his relapse? (As I recall, his relapse in August 1991 was thought to have been related to a too sudden reduction in medication.) In any event, I feel that that sort of information ought to be passed to the St Mungo's staff who have daily supervision of him.

'A further cause of concern is the attitude of the GP. On the morning of May 26th, the date of Jeremy's last admission to the Royal Free, he apparently gave Jeremy two paracetamol and told him he was suffering from 'flu symptoms! When, for the sake of formality and courtesy, I went to see him a couple of hours later to explain that I had spoken to you and you thought it would be best if I brought Jeremy to see you immediately, he would not listen to me, cutting me short with annoyance: "Well, since you've spoken to the consultant already..." Not very reassuring.

'I don't suppose the nursing side of Nicol Ward's operations is your domain exactly, but there too I was somewhat taken aback by the attitude of one of the nurses. She tried to prevent me from seeing Jeremy shortly after you had said it was all right, on the grounds that he had to learn to take responsibility for his own illness (*sic*) and implied that too much involvement with parents was part of the problem. I hope that approach to mental illness is not widespread on the ward: it smacks of RD Laing and *MIND in Camden* (who used to oppose the use of anti-psychotic medication).

'But what concerns me most is the Care Plan: who does what and who tells what to whom. I should be most grateful if you could advise me about this.'

I received no reply.

On August 10th 1993 I wrote again, pointing out that I had received no reply to my previous letter and adding:

'I have in the meantime also contacted the Director of Camden Social Services who delegated the Principal Mental Health Officer, to write to me. He said in effect that Care Programmes were the province of the Health Authority and enclosed a document, which sets out in considerable detail the sort of thing a Care Programme is supposed to entail.

'Yesterday I phoned the Health Authority who told me that they had issued guidelines to the region's hospitals and that, yes,

Care Programme arrangements should conform to the recommendations contained in "The Care Programme Approach" document and I should ask my son's consultant.

'Could you let me know, therefore, how you see the situation?'

What is the Care Plan for my son: letters to the Department of Health and Camden Social Services

On October 7th 1992 I had written to **Virginia Bottomley**, then **Secretary of State for Health**, enclosing a copy of an article I had contributed to the health page of *The Independent*. In the hope of eliciting a response I pointed out that she was related to one of my uncles.

'The most pressing need,' I wrote, 'is for a systematic approach to identifying sufferers and involving them in treatment as early as possible in their illness; for providing carers and relatives with as much information as possible and ensuring that the "authorities" communicate with them; for providing support for sufferers outside hospital, including, most urgently, appropriate sheltered accommodation and sheltered employment, for many are capable of contributing something useful to society.

'If care in the community is to mean anything, it must include at least these basic provisions. At the moment, the situation is terribly confused. You do not know what action to take in a crisis, where to turn for advice and information, what treatments are available, what the likely prognosis is, what contribution the family can or should make to the care of the ill. In the absence of this kind of help, the experience of mental illness is for many an absolute nightmare...'

I received no reply. I wrote again **on February 21**[st] **1993**, with a copy to Glenda Jackson MP. Again I received no reply.

On April 6th **Glenda Jackson received a reply from Tim Yeo, Under Secretary of State for Health**, apologising for the delay in replying to her letter to Virginia Bottomley of February 23rd. It included the following:

'The Government's long standing policy... The Care Programme Approach, operative from April 1991, ... involves drawing up explicit individually tailored care programmes for all in-patients about to be discharged from mental illness hospitals and all new patients accepted by the specialist psychiatric services...'

I received my reply from the Department of Health **on September 7th**. A Mr Dash thanked me for my letter to Virginia Bottomley of April 2nd and said that he had been asked to apologise for the long delay! He then assured me that while there had been difficulties with the Government's new policy, "many of the problems that have arisen in the past will be overcome".

Glenda Jackson's intervention also elicited a response from Camden's **Principal Officer for Mental Health. On May 14th 1993**, referring to the practical difficulties I had mentioned, he said,

'there is no easy way of working with people with acute mental health problems... Camden has a disproportionately large number of diagnosed schizophrenics, in a context of a vast homelessness problem, and the need to be sensitive to the requirements of numerous ethnic groups... Quite clearly there are simply not enough social workers to enable every person suffering from a mental health difficulty (*sic*) to have an allocated worker (a recent survey suggested one person in four in Camden would fit this description) and hence work is allocated on a priority short-term basis with people in an acute phase of their illness. At other times much of the ongoing work has to be undertaken by health service personnel, and voluntary organisations or people's families.'

So, there were not enough social workers. Result: families have to shoulder the burden, in spite of the fact that, in the opinion of some, families are part of the problem. Furthermore, one in four inhabitants of the London Borough of Camden is mad. Odd, that statistic of one-in-four: we will meet it again. And, of course, that continuing obsession with the special requirements of ethnic groups, never clearly defined. (Are Albanians ethnic but Italians not? Are the cultural sensitivities of eastern Turks the same as those of Istanbulis or of Syrians just over the border to the south? We are never told.)

He went on to say that I had touched on a crucial ethical point in my article: 'It is evident to any carer that people suffering from mental illness are seldom, by the nature of their illness, in a state to take an informed decision about what is best for them, nor indeed to assess their own needs in a realistic way.'

'While completely understanding this heartfelt assertion,' he said, 'it is clearly part of an ongoing debate between compulsion and civil liberties... Spokespersons for *MIND* would almost certainly suggest (*sic*) differently... We cannot compel.'

Glenda Jackson had received her reply. I had received nothing, so **on July 12th I wrote to the Director of Camden Social Services**:

'I understand – and this is confirmed by the enclosed copy of a letter from Tim Yeo to Glenda Jackson, my MP – that all psychiatric patients discharged from hospital are meant to have an "individually tailored" Care Plan, which sets out plainly what provisions are to be made for their continuing care outside hospital. I have never seen such a Plan for my son. Is there one? Where is it? Can you procure me a copy of it? And, if there is not one, why is not there one?

'I tried to discover what arrangements were being made for my son this time last year... Nothing remotely resembling a Care Plan was forthcoming. Indeed, one letter (from the Royal Free's Care Management Project; July 31st 1992; copies of correspondence enclosed) appeared to imply that voluntary patients [Jeremy had been admitted without having to be sectioned] were not included in continuing care arrangements...'

This prompted my own reply from the **Principal Officer for Mental Health (on July 23rd 1993)**:

'I am enclosing photocopies of the relevant legislation as it appears that you are confusing the three different processes that could affect the discharge of somebody from psychiatric hospital.'

The three different processes were: Section 117 of the Mental Health Act (1983), Community Care Legislation and the Care Programme Approach. So, in the first case, I had got it wrong because my son, being a voluntary patient and not under Section, was not covered by these after-care arrangements. In the second, the legislation had only come into force on April 1st 1993, therefore any admissions prior to that date were not covered. In the third case, I was told, Tim Yeo had not mentioned an individually tailored "Care Plan", but an individually tailored "Care Programme".

'This is the area where your confusion arises,' the Principal Officer for Mental Health told me and then went on to explain that the care programme does not require a written care plan.

On July 30th I wrote back:

'You are absolutely right... I am confused – totally confused. Neither I nor Jeremy's mother have ever been systematically involved in any sort of consultation regarding his illness and treatment. We have never been offered advice how best to proceed, nor has our advice or help ever been systematically sought by any of the professionals, either in the health or social services, involved in his treatment. Nor have we ever been informed what systematic arrangements have been made for his continuing treatment in the community. And this, in spite of the fact that he has been admitted to hospital five times since 1990.

'Yes, thank goodness, he has a place in a hostel, but that is thanks to the commitment of Jill Gipps whom I took the initiative of contacting during one of his stays in Friern. The system did nothing. He had been allowed to leave a Richmond Fellowship hostel without any further arrangements for his accommodation being made.

'If you knew what we had been through and, Heaven knows, it is fairly small beer compared to some people's experiences, you would not be surprised at our confusion. For instance, Jeremy has just been discharged from the Royal Free after a stay of a month. On the day of his admission, his GP told me he was suffering from 'flu and gave him two paracetamol. The same GP had earlier refused to tell hostel staff what his level of medication was supposed to be, and the Royal Free had not informed them either, in spite of the fact that Jeremy had been resident with them for nearly a year! That has now been rectified.

'Jeremy was in urgent need of admission. It was me who organised it, by contacting the consultant myself. He had suggested referral by the GP. How long would that have taken? Jeremy was raving about going to Libya to talk to Gaddafi and had struck me a hefty straight right on the jaw! When I went, for courtesy's sake, to tell the GP that I was taking Jeremy to hospital, he was totally uncooperative and would not discuss the matter with me, repeating only: "Well, if you've spoken to the consultant already..."

'I will not bore you with the history of the previous three years' confusions. It is more of the same, many times over. That is why I have begun to be rather insistent about a Care Plan. I want to know what arrangements are envisaged for my son. I want to be informed. I want to be told what happens, for example, in a crisis: who takes responsibility for getting Jeremy admitted to hospital? Can we be sure that there will always be a bed? I want to know what level of medication he is on, when it is being reduced and why. I would like someone to discuss other possible treatments with me. Therapy, for example? Would some other drug be more appropriate, less debilitating? How long can he stay in his present hostel? Who will decide when it might be appropriate to try living on his own? What support will he get if he does? What arrangements have been envisaged to help him structure his day, occupy himself? And so on.

'Who is going to tell me these things? Who is one day going to ring up and say, "Mr Salmon, we would like to discuss your son's treatment with you." After all, I see him practically every day. And not once, not once in four years, has anyone made any attempt to involve me or inform me...

'I am not angry with you personally. I am frustrated because I still do not know what exactly the Care Programme Approach means for my son and I do not know who to ask. I should be most grateful if you could tell me.

'I am a reasonably intelligent and well-educated and pugnacious person. What worries me most is, if I can't understand what is supposed to be happening and can't get anybody to tell me, what on earth happens to the thousands of parents, relatives – carers, if you will – who are more easily intimidated than me? An approach to treating the mentally ill which makes so much of involving carers, yet fails to get someone like me to understand what is supposed to be happening seems to me to be pretty seriously flawed.'

His response came **on September 23rd 1993**:

'I am sorry to have been so very long in responding,' he wrote. '... the Care Programme Approach is an initiative involving both Health Service and Social Services and is targeted in particular on those who would otherwise be left "in drift" in a long-stay psychiatric institution. It reflects the Government's intention that the Health Service and Social Services should collaborate to support those who need their care, but leave each agency responsible for its own contribution...'

'Should a crisis occur,' he went on, 'when it appears that Jeremy may need urgent admission to hospital... then the responsibility will lie particularly with his GP and this Department's Approved Social Worker Service...'

'To see the social worker involved with Jeremy last year as "backing off meekly" is to misunderstand their role, and their broader responsibilities.'

In other words, where a social worker's presence is most needed, you can least count on it! And he had himself told Glenda Jackson that 'there is no easy way of working with people with acute mental health problems' (letter of May 14th, above).

What is the Care Plan: letters to the Royal Free Hospital

Not having been able to get much of a response from Camden Social Services, I thought I would try the Health Service. **On August 9th 1993** I phoned the Northeast Thames regional authority and was told that, yes, the Care Programme regulations were now supposed to be operational and that I should speak to my consultant or the hospital's chief executive.

I phoned the hospital and spoke to the Assistant General Manager. He said the hospital was satisfied that my son's discharge plan was in order but they could not guarantee the cooperation of Social Services. There were no formal procedures for involving carers. The patient, if adult, had to request the carers' involvement or at least not object. 'You are obviously a parent who cares very much,' he told me.

Do most parents not care? Is there something peculiar about caring for your children? For this would seem to be the implication.

He was impeccably polite and helpful but getting a definite answer out of him was like trying to trap a drop of mercury. The consultant was responsible but he could not require the co-operation of Social Services. The implementation of the guidelines was a matter for individual hospitals, even individual clinicians.

So, the next day, **August 10th 1993, I wrote to the Chief Executive at the Royal Free**:

'The reason I write to you is that I am trying without much success, to discover precisely what my son's Care Plan or Care Programme is. I am particularly concerned to discover this because there appears to be a large gap between what I understand the Care Programme Approach to entail and what actually happens. The enclosed document, *The Care Programme Approach*, was sent to me by Camden Social Services Principal Mental Health Officer following correspondence with myself and Glenda Jackson MP. I have to say that, although its recommendations appear highly specific, in my experience few of them are implemented.

'In my attempts to discover what my son's Care Programme is I have written to his consultant. He has neither replied to nor acknowledged my letter although a month has now elapsed. I have also written to Camden Social Services whose reply said in effect that Care Programmes were the responsibility of the Health Authority. The Health Authority, however, tell me that they have issued directives to hospitals and that it is up to the hospitals to implement the programme and that, yes, what should happen is pretty much in line with the recommendations set out in *The Care Programme Approach* document and that I should speak to yourself and my son's consultant.

'Yesterday I spoke to your assistant general manager. He was very helpful, but told me in effect that as far as you – that is to say, the Royal Free – were concerned, you had discharged your responsibilities if a patient's discharge was satisfactorily completed. Apart from the fact that the notion of a "satisfactory discharge" seems to me to beg an awful lot of questions, he also said you had no way of effecting a foolproof link between medical needs and those to be met by Social Services.

'What I find puzzling is the fact that none of this seems to tally with the detailed recommendations of *The Care Programme*

Approach, especially in view of the great emphasis that document seems to place on the need for a systematic approach to continuing care of psychiatric patients, and on the need for interprofessional working and the involvement of carers and relatives. What I would like from you is an authoritative account, if you are able to give it, of precisely what the Care Programme Approach means to the Royal Free.

'Camden Social Services Principal Mental Health Officer seemed to be suggesting that my bewilderment was caused by my failure to understand the relevant legislation. That I am confused I readily admit. But what, I ask, is the use of a system that is so woolly and vague and so capable of widely differing interpretation that even a persistent and reasonably intelligent person like myself is quite unable to get a grasp of what is supposed to be happening in the case of my own son? And, if it is indeed true that individual hospitals are responsible for implementing the system, is it not a major failure on your part that you have not been able to inform me? Surely you do not expect carers or relatives, still less the patients who suffer from such a severe and debilitating illness as schizophrenia, to take the initiative of finding out for themselves?

'On more than one occasion it has been more than half suggested to me that since my son is twenty-six, then, of course, that is why I have not been involved in decisions about his care; he would have to ask for his father to be involved. That is a line of argument that I find difficult to describe as anything other than a cop-out.

'I am tired of being shuffled from pillar to post and shall look forward to hearing your view of this whole business at your earliest convenience. And I should, incidentally, be very pleased to meet with you whenever that suits...'

The reply was immediate. My concerns were being investigated by the **General Manager**.

On September 14th 1993 he wrote, reviewing what he called the history of my son's care and finding, unsurprisingly, that everything was as it should be:

'...from the enquiries I have made I believe your son's aftercare to have been properly provided. However,' he added,

'...it is clear from your letters that you are extremely frustrated and dissatisfied with the services which your son has received.'

He suggested that a meeting with himself and my son's consultant 'may be the most productive way forward.'

*

We met, finally, **on November 8th 1993**: the consultant, the general manager, me and a bright young lawyer who worked for the NSF. I had not told the Royal Free that I was bringing her. We just showed up together and I introduced her. Mr Easton was visibly rattled, which was gratifying.

I have no clear recollection of how the meeting went. The general manager blustered about having done everything that should have been done. The consultant was more sympathetic. He apologised for not having involved me more systematically in decisions about what should happen to Jeremy, but said he had not thought it necessary as I involved myself. When, however, we insisted that it was important that the care programme should be "published" in some form since some of the key people involved in Jeremy's care did not seem to be aware that they were even supposed to be part of a team, he promised to call a meeting to which they would all be invited. When I asked whether they would have to attend, he said there was no way of obliging them to, which seemed to be somewhat at odds with the government's pious words about inter-professional working.

We all however received due notification on Royal Free headed paper and the meeting, billed as an Aftercare Review Conference, took place **on November 25th 1993**, three and a half years after my son's first hospital admission. Present were: Jeremy's mother and myself, the GP, Community Psychiatric Nurse, the St Mungo's key-worker plus two social workers, a ward charge nurse plus the consultant and his subordinates. It looked like a true multi-disciplinary meeting, at last.

Not everything went smoothly. I explained why I had made so much fuss about the meeting: that it was important that the arrangements for Jeremy's aftercare should be systematic and public. The nigger in the woodpile, so to speak, turned out to be the GP. In an unpleasant and abrasive manner he said it would be better to leave him out of the discussion as we – I presume he meant me – tended to dramatise the situation, which contributed to Jeremy's illness, and would not listen to him anyway, whereas his own judgement was more objective, more coolly clinical. He said he would not, for example, have recommended Jeremy's last hospital admission, when Jeremy had broken his hostel banisters, landed a straight right on my jaw and was talking of going to see Ghadafi. He himself had diagnosed 'flu and prescribed two paracetamol, His view was that Jeremy should be given his medication by long-lasting depot injection, something which Jeremy had always refused, although now this is how he takes his medication and it does indeed seem to be effective. In that sense the GP was right, but the way he put it made it sound as if he believed that "what these people need" is to be "drugged up" willy-nilly so that they did not cause trouble.

Minutes were taken, although they did not record the unhelpful and aggressive attitude of the GP. Seven recommendations were made, mainly to do with the different levels of responsibility for supervising Jeremy's health: who would alert whom. It was agreed that the situation should be reviewed every three months and that all this would be put into writing.

I walked home with the St Mungo's key-worker. He told me it was the first time he had met the GP, even though they worked scarcely ten minutes' walk from each other. Given the doctor's attitude, this was not surprising but it did not augur well for the trouble-free running of a system of care for the mentally ill in which, then as now, the GP/Primary Care Team was supposed to be the lynch-pin, the first line of defence. He also said that he had never heard of any other hostel resident getting this kind of attention from the powers-that-be: quite simply they did not have anyone to fight their corner.

That was 1993.

The arrangements agreed upon at this meeting worked and were adhered to for a while, though lapsed eventually. I emphasise the date because now it is 2008. My son is much better at the moment, thank God. Yet still, fifteen years down the line, it is not absolutely clear what his Care Plan is; there are still lapses in communication. In the last three months, for instance, there have been two changes of care co-ordinator, as the person with front-line responsibility for him is now called. On neither occasion have I been officially notified.

Chapter Five
Living Alone

Reading through all this correspondence, re-awakening the memory of half-forgotten names and conversations, I get the impression that schizophrenia must have filled all the space in my life.

Certainly, it filled a lot. Jeremy was only two streets away and would come round frequently, always unannounced. He still does that: I may be in the middle of something. I could say, no, I'm busy – the setting boundaries school of relations. I think that is baloney, especially when it is your own child who is in need, a need so much greater than that most of us ever have to face. I let him in.

He would make cups of tea, often four or five in succession, and never drink any of them or only half: I would find them scattered about the house after he had left. The same with fags: endless roll-ups that went out, that had to be re-lit, that went out. His fingers were yellow-black with tobacco. And the cans of beer: never so much that he was drunk, but more than was good to combine with the medication he was taking. I often failed but always tried not to comment, not always to say, 'Oh, don't smoke any more. You should try to cut down. Don't have another beer. Your hair is getting a bit long. When did you last have a haircut? We could go together.' So that everything seemed a criticism, although I only spoke out of concern, anxiety. I did not want him to look strange. He often smelt of tobacco and beer. I did not want people to shy away from him. He's a nutter. That dreaded reaction.

I could no more have turned him away than cut off my own arm, although being with him was often nerve-wracking. His moods were so volatile. If I pointed out, as he made his third cup of tea, that there were already two un-drunk ones on the table, if I chose the wrong moment (and how could you ever know when the right one was?) to suggest he might go down to the NSF project at King's Cross... he was always talking about a job, about working. Whenever anyone asked what he needed, it was never medication; if anything, it was the medication that was preventing him from getting a job. If you said the wrong thing the wrong way at the wrong time, he could fly off the handle. No matter how I tried to help, no matter how I tried to make things better, there was nothing I could do.

I remembered my mother's story of how when I was little and was taken for a walk in my pram they used to run ahead and stand the dead blackbirds up so I would not be upset. I wanted to stand the dead blackbirds up for my son and I could not. My friend Geoff would remind me: he loves you, he admires you, he just needs you to be there, so he can come round. Don't pay any attention to the moods, the humours.

I felt so sorry for him. An abiding image of him: I stand in my doorway watching him walk off down the street, slightly stooping, unkempt, his jeans hanging off his bum, his ancient leather jacket hunched, one hand held low down at his side, the fingers slightly splayed and stretched in an awkward-looking, unnatural posture – so often the give-away sign of someone on anti-psychotic medication. And my heart would ache, would break, really. He looked so alone, so isolated. It brought tears to my eyes. I had to try not to watch him go, to say goodbye at the door, in the house.

Not that he was always unkempt. Sometimes he would be freshly shaved, washed and brushed, cheerful; and he looked his old handsome self and my hopes would rise again. He can be all right, he will be all right. If only...

Every time I glimpsed his old pre-illness self I would seize eagerly on the moment, suggesting courses... You could easily do French; after all, you speak pretty well already. Or take up Greek: you have not really forgotten that. Or gardening projects... I visited an NSF gardening project in Faversham where five or six people seemed to have found real sanctuary and sustenance and

Geoff knew someone who had worked on the Mencap garden by the canal bridge at Westbourne Park. Sometimes I would ask him to explain some point of science, something to do with biology, say, or chemistry and when he did so, lucidly and simply, I would feel ridiculously proud and reassure myself that underneath he was all right, his brain still functioned normally, his intelligence was still there.

I swung between extreme anxiety and clutching at straws, my ear finely tuned to the nuances of tone and timbre in his voice, my eyes searching his gaze, scrutinising his face, straining to read his mood, gauge how he was. I was always looking for grounds for hope. I wanted to believe. His mother, on the other hand, was always gloomy about his prospects, finding him aggressive, unhappy and difficult. I could never get her to say that she found him well. And he has been well. There are times when he is well. Is she right? Am I deluding myself? Is the situation really desperate, without any hope or any redeeming element?

I go away. I go away on research trips to France for the Rough Guide. Sometimes I am away for several weeks. I go to Greece, to the mountains. It is my work. It is also my lifeline. Geoff tells me: if you fall apart, what use are you going to be to Jeremy? You have got to keep your own life going. I assuage my guilt with that thought. Also I know it to be true. I have seen what happens to people – nearly always mothers – who sacrifice their own lives entirely to caring for a child, a husband, sometimes both: worn out, nothing but a rag of life left.

I try to phone every day or every other day when I am away. Jeremy does not like it when I go away and I generally get punished for it: he will not speak to me for a few days before I leave and after I get back. I am anxious when I call, straining to understand how he is; and generally things are okay. Sometimes he says he misses me and occasionally breaks down in tears and then I am racked: I feel hopeless and helpless.

*

Around this time I tried to get regular employment. The occasional painting and decorating that I used to do with Geoff was not really enough. I saw an advertisement for an English language teacher in Hampstead and applied. I was asked to come for an interview. It was only when I got there that I realised it was the same "school" I had had a temporary post with in the first year of Jeremy's illness, when I had stood in for a teacher who was having a baby and they would not re-employ me for a second term because some of the students had complained about me! The premises were different but I recognised the fur-coated woman who interviewed me. Luckily she did not recognise me. I had not bothered to prepare for the interview. I had been teaching for years. I had been head of department several times. I knew what I was doing.

It turned out to be the most embarrassing and humiliating interview I ever had. I was interviewed by two people. The questions were asked by the fur-coated owner of the school whose only professional qualification was as a nurse. She asked me, reasonably enough, how I would go about teaching au pair girls from different language backgrounds. For some reason I was completely taken aback. I hummed and hawed a bit about direct method and my mind went blank. I could not think of anything to say. I felt a deep blush creeping up my neck and face. She asked me what books I would use. I could not remember the name of a single course book I had ever seen. Somewhat exasperated she asked what books I had used in my last job. I could not remember anything except LG Alexander, a rather old-fashioned course written by a Greek Cypriot, who once waited an extra day in a Greek mountain village just to meet me. Perhaps I should have told that story; a man who had read my book and waited in order to meet me... But I did not have the presence of mind. I sat there, tongue-tied and embarrassed, while this fur-clad nurse looked at me with contempt, as if I were a rather shabby con man caught *in flagrante.* A pervert whose elaborate wheeze for getting close to au pair girls had been ingloriously exposed.

Rather than suffer the further humiliation of having her terminate the interview, I stood up, muttering something about there not being much point in pursuing this any further and, gathering, as it were, my dignity about me, headed confidently for the door, opened it and to my horror found myself looking into the dark interior of a cupboard. I turned back to the room. I do not remember whether I saw the real door first or whether the fur coat had to point it out to me. I who had been head of GCE at Athens College, head of English in grammar schools and comprehensives, the author of books, I who had been on TV and radio... Not only could I not get through an interview with a nurse for a part-time job teaching English to au pair girls, I could not even find the door I had come in by! A bad moment.

It was at this time also that I began to house-hunt, looking for a flat to buy with the money my Greek mother-in-law had so generously given me. I wanted to tell Jeremy about it, to give him something to look forward to, to give him hope: the promise of a place of his own, a home, instead of the indefinite prospect of life in institutions or public housing. At the same time I was afraid of encouraging him to undertake something he could not manage, of having him put pressure on me to let him live in the place before he was ready. The absolute priority was to stay within the catchment area of the Royal Free.

I saw places that were far from shops, places where the access was much too communal, would bring you into too close contact with the neighbours, places on top floors or with an obviously tempting drop from a window. I saw places that could have been nice – I believe in the therapeutic power of the beauty of a place: by that I mean its vibe, its feel, quite as much as design or architectural merit – but had been spoilt by conversion, by the developer's conventional ideas about the deployment of space and his greedy desire to cram as many marketable living units into his property as possible. The obviously attractive and suitable places were always just out of reach financially.

I settled in the end on a place in Kilburn, just the right side of the High Road for the Royal Free. It had been newly converted, in a cheap and horrible manner, the walls covered with a pink paper decorated with a kind of rubberised white motif in semi-relief; you could pinch the white bits, lift them up and release them so that they snapped back into place like elastic. And the brand new carpet was made of a synthetic fibre that created an effect to the touch similar to that created aurally by a fingernail screeching on a blackboard. But the flat was on a top floor with a living room and bedroom facing due south, catching every bit of light and ray of sunshine. It had a spacious kitchen and another small room looking over some rooftops to the Jubilee Line, so you saw the trains slide by 100m away, but silently because of the double-glazing. The bathroom was windowless, but I decided that did not matter too much. There was a big loft area. And the stairs leading up to it from the ground were basically mine.

The bottom two floors were a business run by some elderly Czech wartime refugees, so no sound from below outside business hours. Their entrance was on the main street. Ours was from a quiet cul-de-sac at the back, through a door into a little courtyard garden that served three other small flats, then through a second door to our stairs. The surrounding area was a little insalubrious, but respectable and the approaches private and safe. Airy and light, the flat had a good feel to it. It had been on the market for a while, I imagine, because the configuration of space that suited us did not suit more normal customers, and it was relatively cheap, probably for the same reason, which would leave enough money spare to do it up and furnish it.

I had never done anything like this before and I was apprehensive. I showed Geoff and another friend, who had a schizophrenic son. They both thought it was right and so I bought it. Geoff said he would help me fix it as I had lodged and fed him for so long. We worked at it for weeks, finding the usual mess and botch that builders leave: areas of unstable plaster hidden behind the hideous rubberised paper – probably nothing else would have held it in place; old pipes and bricks stuffed out of the way under the floorboards. Jeremy came and kept us company while we worked. He sat cross-legged and motionless on the floor. He had become interested in Buddhism and silent contemplation in the lotus position seemed to suit his humour. One day, after he had left, I found an off-cut of timber on which he had written in a neat, tight hand: "May the grain in this wood be blessed." I have kept it. Sometimes, for an hour or two, he would help with the painting.

Then Geoff vanished on one of his amorous adventures and I had to finish the flat alone. I have never liked working in Jeremy's flats on my own. I am always filled with apprehension when preparing them for his arrival and gloom when tidying up after he has had to leave. I feel very lonely.

It was obvious that for the moment Jeremy was not going to be able to live in the flat, so I would have to let it. One day I had a brainwave. There was a nice, tidy, well-organised girl living on her own with a baby in one of the other small flats on the courtyard, and she had to move. I asked her if she would like to rent my place. She came and had a look and said that she would like to but would have to arrange for Housing Benefit. And so it came about.

*

Jeremy was not well at this time. He hated the hostel. His medication did not seem to be very effective. He was taking Stellazine pills and probably missing days here and there, though he always denied it. My biggest fear was that he would be run over. He had bought an old bike, which he rode as if there were no other traffic on the street. He gave no hand signals and wobbled about the roadway apparently oblivious.

An old friend who is an eminent scientist was living nearby at the time. With a research partner he had developed a vaccine, *mycobacterium vaccae*, primarily as a treatment for tuberculosis. One day we met in the street and he asked me about my son. He was in the process of setting up a bio-tech company to develop this discovery and he started telling me about it. He told me that in the course of tests for this treatment in various parts of the world some unexpected results had been found. His research partner had noticed that in some patients suffering from TB but also presenting with symptoms of schizophrenia their schizophrenia had appeared to improve. The vaccine works, crudely put, by switching off the body's auto-immune system and there was a belief, discredited now but based largely, I believe, on research carried out in the USSR, that schizophrenia might be an auto-immune disease.

My friend's research partner had a son who suffered from schizophrenia and he, as well as one or two others, had been treated with injections of this vaccine for some time with apparently quite positive results. My friend thought it was worth trying and assured me that there could not be any adverse effects.

I was excited. The partner was a firm believer in the positive effects of the treatment. I told my NSF group about it and we got him to come and talk to us. Obviously, it was not a replacement for standard anti-psychotic medication. The research evidence was encouraging. There did not appear to be any danger. Why not give it a try, as I had the luck to have access to it? I told Jeremy's consultant. He discussed the matter with my friends and gave his consent. Jeremy himself agreed and he had his first shot.

Clutching at straws, some might say. Placebo effect, some might say, wishful thinking... But I saw a marked improvement in my son's health within a very few days. I have in front of me the letter I wrote to the consultant at the end of May 1994: 'A word to let you know how Jeremy is now that six weeks have elapsed since he received his first shot of Dr S's vaccine... A marked improvement was evident within ten days and has been maintained, with perhaps one slight hiccough, ever since. How has it manifested itself?

'First of all, my parent's instinct about my child's health told me that there had been a significant shift. His eyes looked clearer. Some of the drawn look went from his face. I no longer felt so on edge in his presence, as if anything might happen at any moment. His talk became more lucid and rational; that characteristic discourse that is neither quite sense nor quite nonsense has almost completely disappeared. I can address any subject with him, including his illness and other matters he finds awkward and would formerly evade by leaving the room or falling silent.

'More specifically, he came all the way to Chiswick several days running to help me with a painting job I was doing. Some days he came by public transport, something he would not have attempted a couple of months ago. Other days he came with me, which meant being at my door at 6.30am. For the last week he has been staying with me. I have felt no unease or anxiety. He has sat down to meals and finished them with me. He has taken some interest in my life. We have been able to hold a sensible conversation. He has sat all day at his computer typing up his diary of the years since his illness. He has started a sort of graduate back-to-work course, which involves getting himself to Old Street and mixing with fellow-students all day.

'He is not 100% his old self and there have been spasmodic attempts in the past to embark on courses. But there is a real difference about him this time, which others who know him well have remarked on...

'All this to say: I don't want to proclaim a miracle and I keep my fingers tightly crossed, but there is no doubt in my mind that since he had Dr S's injection something quite dramatic has happened. He is more normal, more himself than at any time in the five years since he first became ill. Whether or not this is due to the injection... But Dr S tells me this is very much the pattern they have come to expect with the few patients who have been treated in this way...'

My letter crossed in the post with one from the consultant telling me that there were problems at the hostel and that Jeremy had stopped attending outpatient appointments at the hospital and was becoming reluctant to take his medication. Was the experiment with *mycobacterium vaccae* the cause, at least in part, of his reluctance to take regular medication? Was I being over-optimistic, merely deceiving myself into seeing the result that I so longed for? Was I so partisan on my son's behalf that I refused to accept the reality of his condition and his behaviour in favour of what I wished to be the case? No doubt there were those who thought so.

There was no satisfactory conclusion to Jeremy's encounter with *mycobacterium vaccae*. He had a total of three, possibly four, injections before refusing to have any more. None of the subsequent ones produced quite such a dramatic change as the first, but I remain convinced that did something and that that something was good. But that was the end of that. Another "if only", another wild grasp at a "miracle" came to nothing. And yet, was it such a crazy idea? That same friend told me today, fifteen and more years later, that a paper in the current issue of the journal *Neuroscience* shows how *mycobacterium vaccae* administered to mice does indeed affect the central nervous system!

*

Jeremy so hated the hostel that he had begun to ask about "his" flat. When the tenant said she would be leaving in the autumn, I told him he could move in. I was not popular with the hospital or the social workers. Georgie Hardie, one of the few social workers assigned to Jeremy, whom I really trusted, wrote to tell me, 'I do not need to remind you that the view of all the professionals at the meeting when you first told us of the decision for Jeremy to move out from St Mungo's was that at the moment the hostel is felt to be the most appropriate and supportive setting for him'.

I was very apprehensive about his move. I was afraid he would be lonely, I was afraid he would not feed himself properly, I was afraid the flat would get into a terrible mess. Georgie Hardie's letter rattled me. But I was also afraid of what might happen if the hostel decided they could not cope with him. Then where would he go? You heard tales of people ending up in cheap bed and breakfast in King's Cross. And Jeremy wanted to try. I thought the sense of having his own place, of having a home that was his, with his things, his furniture, his books, his music, a place that others could not enter, might in itself be therapeutic.

I had already checked that the Council were happy to pay Housing Benefit to cover the rent. They had come round to have a look at the place, decided it was bigger than absolutely necessary for one person and settled on a sum that they were prepared to pay. That was okay with me.

On October 27th 1994 we had a Care Plan review meeting. Probably, by now, I should not have been surprised, but I only received notice of the meeting from the Royal Free two days after the event. A letter from Georgie Hardie containing potentially crucial and, as it turned out, completely erroneous information provided by a DSS Residential Care Manager to the effect that the Council were most unlikely to agree to pay Housing Benefit as I, a relative, was to be my son's landlord, also arrived after the event. I protested. The hospital once again found that it had followed procedures entirely correctly and was itself in no way to blame. As to the Social Worker, she was an employee of Camden Social Services and "therefore falls outside our remit". Not apparently noticing any irony, they also averred that "it is of great importance that carers are involved as much as possible in these situations (*sic*)".

November 1st was the day appointed for Jeremy's move. He told the meeting he was confident about the move but would like to stop taking medication because he wanted to look for a job.

The consultant told him that, on the contrary, if he was thinking in terms of a job taking medication would be all the more important.

It was distressing to hear Jeremy talk like this. You could say it was natural for a young and vigorous man to want to be out in the world, working, forging a life for himself; that is what his friends and contemporaries were doing. But did he not know, really not understand, that in his current condition it would have been impossible to find a job, that no employer would have him or that, even if he were to find a job, he would not be able to do it? It was particularly distressing, as well as a little alarming, to see him so unrealistic about his situation, now, as he was about to try living on his own.

His move was very thoroughly prepared: outpatient appointments, a social worker, a CPN, a plan for action if he were to relapse, benefits... Georgie Hardie was to make a Care Needs Assessment. (I was given a copy of a paper about this time showing that authorities were being asked to avoid identifying needs that could not be met!) Everything seemed to be in place. The bed was made, his books were on the shelves, his pictures on the walls.

I do not know what he was feeling but I was extremely anxious the day I drove him round to begin his new life. And in an important sense it was a new life, I believe, in spite of the difficulties and risks. He was twenty-eight. If nothing else had turned out as he would have wished, at least he had his own home.

I don't remember how long I stayed before leaving him to spend his first night alone in the flat. In physical terms it was not far: two stops on the Tube, ten or twelve minutes by car or on my bike. There was another kind of distance involved. He was quite frightened, I think, and so was I. Hostels were hateful to him: 'surrounded by all those nutters, Dad.' But they were society. They were a kind of community, albeit unwilling; the experience of nuttiness was itself an important thing to have in common. Whereas here, isolated behind your own front door, among neighbours who went about ordinary lives, regulated and given meaning by the – for him unattainable – routines of work, family life, daily chores... Cut off from the workaday world of companionship and shared experience by a routine so different, cut off even more by the illness itself, whose most devastating symptom in Jeremy's case has always been paranoia, that deep suspicion of all other people which makes even the limited human contact of a transaction over a shop counter an ordeal, a skirmish with the most dangerous and threatening of enemies.

I cannot really imagine what it was like for him. In fact I prefer not to try; it makes me too unhappy. I try to take comfort in what I see: a person, who in spite of everything is still there, still fighting, still surviving.

God knows what he went through that first night, once the door closed behind me. Perhaps he was already so used to the self-absorption, the turned-inwardness that the illness forces on you, that he felt no different from any other night. He survived it. I do not remember what he said. We spoke on the phone, usually several times a day. When he was not well, he would put the phone down or leave me horrible messages, abusive and crazy. I saw him frequently. He never made mention of the nasty messages he had left. I would cycle over, my heart always in my mouth. The flat, so carefully and lovingly prepared for him, quickly became a mess: cigarette burns in the carpet, on the edges of the bookshelves or the kitchen worktops, from the endless fag-ends balanced there and left to burn out. There were burns in the sheets, but miraculously he never set fire to himself. There were papers all over the floor, the endless notes and jottings that he made, that make up his book, letters neatly addressed but mostly unsent; plates of food, partly eaten, the leftovers set hard; ash on his sofa, Rizla papers in the bed sheets, beer cans, some empty, some not, so that when you picked them up to throw them away stale beer spilled.

But these were my worries. In spite of my awful imaginings, he seemed to manage. He liked being in the flat and he did not like it – still does not – if I attempted to "clear up" too often. 'I want to see you, Dad,' he says. 'I don't want to spend time with a maid.'

What did he do all day? There were shops nearby. Lord knows what he ate, but he did not have far to go to do his shopping: fags, beer and pasta mainly. And there were plenty of take-away places. There was a rather strange pub he used to frequent and tell me tales of some of the people he met there. Most unsuitable, was my parental reaction, though uncharacteristically I kept it to myself. At least it was company.

He read. He wrote. He meditated. Often when I rang up he would say he was meditating. He bought books about Buddhism and there were often Buddhist Society leaflets strewn about the flat. I think it must have had a beneficent influence: he could not do the not-drinking, but living in the present, accepting – that, I think, helped.

And then there was the girlfriend, the Korean girl he had met in hospital. She was not well either, but she was quiet and amenable, in fact seemed a little doped by her medication. She even managed a job of some kind for a while, working with fellow Koreans – they may have been relatives and made allowances. She worked on a computer, but was very troubled by it; her version of hearing voices was believing that computers and television sets could see into her mind and control her. Often she would ask whether it were true that computers could read what was going on in your mind. She was frightened. Although she was much easier to deal with than Jeremy, I think that in many ways she was crazier. She was a compulsive hand-washer, always trying to cleanse herself.

She was good for Jeremy. She would stay over sometimes for two or three days, when her mother was away. Her mother did not like her daughter's association with Jeremy and did her best to obstruct it. She was a petite, pretty woman, apparently a skilled dressmaker. She had an Englishman in tow; I believe they were married although they did not appear to live together. The daughter's father, back in Korea, had suffered from schizophrenia and made life very difficult for them, which was, I think, the reason they had left. They came to see me once, the mother and the English husband. By a strange coincidence he had taught in an art school where my friend Geoff had been a student. They came to see me in an attempt to get me to stop Jeremy seeing the daughter, which I refused to do. I saw no reason why these two kids should not enjoy the solace of a relationship together. I think my nose was also put rather out of joint by the implication that somehow my son was not good enough for her daughter.

Things seemed to be going fairly well in the flat for the first couple of months. Jeremy took his medication, kept his Outpatient appointments, kept in touch with his Social Worker. He went down to the NSF project at King's Cross and made some moves to get involved in other activities, though he never really followed any of these initiatives up. He never seemed to be able or even perhaps to want to make any relationships that could help to fill that void of loneliness or draw him into some continuing shared activity that might begin to bring some meaning, some purpose to his existence.

Then quite suddenly he began to deteriorate. When that happens he stops shaving. His hair gets wild and tangled. He does not change his clothes. He began to complain about the neighbours making a noise. He could hear them talking, he said. I had never heard anyone talking or making any other kind of noise in all the time I had spent working in the flat. There were no neighbours underneath. The only people you might have heard were in the flat at the top of the adjacent building, on the other side of his bedroom wall. But it was not just the sound of their voices that bothered him; in some way their talking was related to him, that was what bothered him. They were this, they were that; he eff-ed and blinded about them. It has become such a common pattern over the years that I am sure neighbours' voices are in fact an embodiment of the voices that he hears in his own head.

Late one January evening he rang me in real distress. He made little sense on the phone and was clearly frightened. I said, 'I'm coming.' I got in the car and was there in ten minutes. My whole body was on crisis alert. On my way to school once I saw a dog react to the sudden realisation that a car was upon him: a matter of life and death. Transfixed, transformed by fear, he became fear; he became muscle, unthinking reflex – his whole body shrank and bunched, contracted into a coil occupying perhaps half the space he would normally occupy, until, by now almost under the front bumper of the approaching car, he uncoiled, the coiled body released itself and he sprang clear. I felt a bit like that; all my faculties shut down except those required to deal with the crisis. Everything concentrated. I think I let out some terrible sobs and groans on the way; that seems to clear all extraneous, superfluous obstacles to concentration. Into the courtyard, through the downstairs door – ajar as so often (I always worried he would leave everything open and unlocked one day and find everything gone) – and up the stairs. 'It's me,' I said, pushing open the unlocked front door to the flat and taking the last flight of stairs two at a time, wholly concentrated now on what I was going to find.

All the lights were on. The radiators were on. Everything was in a mess. He was in the bedroom, on his feet, in his shirt and underpants, bedclothes strewn about wildly, his eyes wild. There was a turd on the floor among the sheets. He was so ashamed and distressed. 'It does not matter, love. Come on. Let's go. You can't stay here.'

I cannot remember exactly what I did. I think I got him to put his trousers on, turned the lights off and left, taking him with me. I do not remember whether we spent the night at my house or went straight to the Royal Free. I think we went straight to the hospital. The "Section" notice is dated February 2nd 1995.

When he is in hospital life shifts a gear. He is safe at least. The outer rings of fortification can be left unmanned for a while. Of course his freedom is curtailed, especially when he is on "Section", but for me that is a relief. Anxiety does not go away. There are almost daily visits to the hospital. They are nearly always painful: because it is painful to see him ill and know there is no cure; because the physical conditions of living are so deplorable – no privacy, the forced association with all degrees of lunacy; the sight of your child brought, in a way, so low. But the first line of defence, the ensuring of his actual physical safety, is someone else's responsibility.

Camilla had come to see me at Christmas. I took her to meet my parents. For the first time in my life my mother actually liked and approved of a woman I brought home. She even asked Camilla to marry me!

With Jeremy safe in hospital I went to California to see her. She told me this morning, when I asked about the dates of our various meetings, that she had thought I was coming to ask her to marry me and was very disappointed when I did not! I did feel safe with her. We decided that she would leave her job and flat and come and live with me in London in May. I had told her of course about Jeremy and what a large part he played in my life: that his illness was a responsibility that I could never abandon. I warned her too that he could be very jealous of my interest in or contact with other people. She accepted that and always has. Indeed I am sure I could not have borne that responsibility with such fortitude or survived it so relatively unscathed without her support.

Once he was safely in hospital I went back to the flat the next day to collect some things for him, his washing things, a few spare clothes. I hate going into his flat when he is in hospital. It is partly that the mess is such a powerful and poignant reminder of the extent to which he cannot do all those things that, as we grow up, we expect to take in our stride in our lives and that he too expected to take in his stride and that I expected him to be able to take in his stride, just like everybody else, before anything went wrong. Things so ordinary that in fact one does not even think about them as being part of the difficulties of life as an adult. But, more than that, it is his absence, the plain fact of his not being there that hurts so much, that fills me with loneliness and dread, terror even: how are we going to get through this? The letters that he writes, to me, to his mother, to his sister, to the consultant, to his granny: the neatly addressed envelopes, stamped, lie about all over the floor and are never sent – better often that they should not be, for when he is not well they can be wild and abusive. The sheets of paper covered with notes, doggerel, poems, wild sometimes, poetic sometimes, and, worst, deeply moving because expressive of such loneliness, isolation and frustration. I pick them up, try to arrange them, impose some order, put them somewhere safe. I clean behind and under things, picking up endless fag-ends, emptying overflowing ashtrays, collecting beer cans. There are piles of washing up, cups and glasses partly filled with unidentifiable liquid capped by lids of strange-coloured growth. I feel unbearably lonely as I do it, sick in the pit of my stomach, filled with a melancholy that hurts me physically. How am I going to get through this? And I sob and groan and lament aloud to myself. How could anything be as cruel and unfair as this? How could anyone do such a thing to my son, my beautiful cherished boy?

And then the place is clean again. The windows sparkle. I leave them open for a day or two. The sun streams in, whenever it gets the chance. The place smells fresh again. I get the chance to paint the stairs white, something I had been meaning to do ever since my earlier tenant first moved in. White lifts the spirit. And I get rid of the rest of that horrible synthetic carpet that originally carpeted the whole flat and sets your teeth on edge when you touch it. That makes the place brighter too.

I go to the local glazier. I have known them for years. They make some secondary glazing units for me, to reduce the traffic noise in Jeremy's bedroom. One of the brothers comes round to fit them. I tell him about Jeremy and he tells me that his son had schizophrenia, but disappeared three years ago and had not been seen or heard of since. That gives you pause. I interviewed a well-known writer once whose son had schizophrenia. He was a gentle boy, easy to get on with, she said. He had lived at home for much of his illness. His torment was believing that a gang of Nigerians had infected his blood and were trying to poison him. He was about thirty, if I remember, when he told his mother he wanted to go and live in a hostel. He did so, but disappeared after a few months and no one knew what had happened to him until, some eighteen months later, his mother received a call from Wapping river police...

I suppose we all live with the fear of some such awfulness at the back of our minds. That is an absence I do not think I could bear, although sometimes you wonder whether death would not be a merciful release.

But I have tidied the flat, made things better. I have done something. Hope comes again. It has to. This is just a relapse, just a temporary thing. He always gets better. We'll make a fresh start...

Perhaps I am just standing up dead blackbirds. What else can we do? Do nothing at all? That is not an option.

My mother does the same. She has found a shop in Hampstead through her sister that will deliver a basket of fruit to my son's flat when she asks them to. About the most expensive way of doing it, I am sure, but when it is a question of giving pleasure to others, making them better, nothing will stand in Mum's way. She is standing up blackbirds too, and I say nothing. I think she has more or less resigned herself to the fact that Jeremy is ill and there is nothing anyone can do about that. It is not any longer my fault for going off with unsuitable women!

While Jeremy was in hospital this time Georgie Hardie did a comprehensive assessment of his needs – her view, his view and his parents'. The upshot? That the main problems he faced were isolation and loneliness and a lack of motivation so that it was difficult for him to find any meaningful activity and follow it up. That he found relations with other people difficult and was rather fearful of them to the point where, when not well, he could hardly bring himself to leave the house. He himself said that he was lonely and felt as if he were always waiting for someone. She proposed that he needed someone to go in and clean for him and generally support and encourage him in finding some way of occupying himself and of broadening the network of people he was engaged with. She suggested too that he might need some help in dealing with his finances.

We are talking about 1995. It is now 2008. None of these things has ever happened. Social workers and CPNs have come and gone, but no one has ever been assigned to clean for him or even to help him clean his flat. Georgie Hardie suggested that he might need access to the Meals on Wheels freezer service. We have never heard a word about that. He has actually always managed his money pretty sensibly, but the complicated bureaucratic Benefits system that gives him his money... he has never received any help with that, although one might have thought that should be a priority.

He is difficult, my son, that goes without saying. But where is the use of a system that in thirteen years has not been able to tackle any of his central needs, even the straightforward practical ones like benefits and prescriptions?

Jeremy's discharge must have taken place around the end of April, beginning of May. He went back to his flat, which he much preferred to St Mungo's in spite of the difficulties, he told

Georgie Hardie. And what did he do? He started organising a trip to Thailand! It was all to do with his interest in Buddhism. I tried to talk him out of it. 'It is so far away. Why don't you start with a journey to somewhere nearer home? Why don't you go to France where we have family?'

I had nightmares about trying to get him out of a Thai jail if anything went wrong, if someone, for instance, were to say or do anything that provoked his anger, never mind the dangers of drug plants. I was particularly worried about Thailand because a friend had had to fly there to rescue her schizophrenic daughter, not because she got into any trouble, but because she woke up one morning to find the alcoholic boyfriend she had travelled out with dead in bed beside her.

Nothing however seemed to deter him. Without telling him I wrote to the company he was planning to travel with and told them he was not well. I also warned his consultant who said that he would have him 'sectioned' if he tried to go. The kind of thing that would have the politically correct rights organisations shrieking outrage! So easy and gratifying to promote virtue and prescribe correct behaviour for others when there is not the slightest chance you will have to live with the consequences yourself!

I forget exactly how this enterprise ended, whether or not the company turned him down on the evidence of what I had told them. But he did not go. By way of consolation I suggested we went to France and Belgium, just the two of us. We took tents. We camped the first night in a small campsite near the hill that the Duke of York marched so vainly up and down. The next day we went to Mons and Ypres and looked at the war memorials. I have a photo of him looking pale. Then we went to Bruges. We found somewhere to stay, parked our luggage and set off to walk around the town.

I do not know what happened. There was some kind of disagreement. I tried to paper over it and he thumped me in the street. 'In that case you can look after yourself,' I said and flounced off. After a couple of hundred yards I repented. I can't leave him like that. I turned back and found him pretty much where I had left him. 'Come on, honey, let's be friends. I don't want to fight. We are supposed to be having a holiday.' He said he was sorry and we went back to our little hotel. We had a discussion about what we were going to do. He said he would rather go home. I said, 'Well, let's wait till the morning and see how we feel then.' He did not want to go out again, so we ate some take-away and went to bed. In the morning we turned for home. He did say with a wry smile that it was a good thing he was not in Thailand.

Reason, reason... there is no reason why it should not work, why we should not be able to go on holiday together, to go at least on a short journey. We get on well together. I love him, he loves me. But reason has nothing to do with it. I am standing up blackbirds again.

Chapter Six
Contracts And Other Ploys

To my regret, Georgie Hardie left and was replaced by a student social worker. She was both very nice and very pretty, which gave her a certain interest in Jeremy's eyes, but being a student she was not likely to be long in her post. And she was not: after five or six months she was gone, just as we were beginning to establish some kind of relationship and a degree of trust. I do not remember anything about her replacement nor how long she lasted. In due course her place was taken by a male community psychiatric nurse (CPN) whom Jeremy did not like and would not co-operate with.

So began a period of some six years during which Jeremy had next to no contact with any social worker or community psychiatric nurse. His consultant retired. After the rocky start to our relationship, I had come to like and appreciate and rely on him. I knew that I could go directly to him in a crisis and that he would always take Jeremy into hospital if necessary. I felt very exposed and vulnerable when he left.

One of the last ploys we tried together was getting Jeremy to sign a contract. It was an idea I had picked up from my French psychiatrist cousins who told me that when they discharged a patient they signed a contract with him: he undertook to take his medication, turn up for outpatient appointments and so forth on pain of being recalled to hospital if he defaulted. It was an innovation that I thought might be worth trying with Jeremy and the consultant was game as ever. So Jeremy signed up to visiting a day centre three times a week; allowing a support group worker to visit him at home to help with the upkeep and maintenance of his flat; co-operating with his social worker and CPN and attending meetings; taking his medication regularly and attending Outpatients at the hospital. The social worker signed, I signed, his mum signed, the professor signed. The sanction was that, if he defaulted, I would not renew the lease on the flat after March 1996 and he would have to move into sheltered accommodation.

Things must have gone relatively well to start with. I have in front of me the minutes of a review meeting held in April: 'It was felt generally that things were going well...although Jeremy has reservations about using the ... Day Centre.' It was agreed that I would renew the lease on the flat for another six months and the various other conditions would continue to apply. I see that it was also agreed that the CPN would take a "back seat role" if Jeremy 'was in contact with other services.'

And there of course was the rub. There the rub has always been. Contact. Contact with other people, people other than his mother and me.

There was the girlfriend. There were periods when they saw a lot of each other, although it was never enough for Jeremy. She had some kind of job for a while and she also had to escape from her mother who did everything possible to prevent her seeing Jeremy. I know he was sometimes aggressive with her, but they were very comfortable together and comfortable with my wife and me. They would turn up at our door, usually unannounced, drink cups of tea and smoke endlessly. She would ask for the n-th time whether I thought the computers were reading her thoughts. They never stayed long.

They were good for each other – and for my confidence: I felt more secure knowing that Jeremy had a real friend in her. She spurred him to be adventurous. He organised a stay for them both at an NSF respite hotel in the New Forest. On another occasion they rented a car, in Bristol, I think it was, although I do not remember what they were doing there, and drove it to Hereford to see my parents. The thought of them driving terrified my mother and I think it had frightened Jeremy too, as it was several years since he had last driven, so my mother arranged for the car hire company to send one of their employees to fetch the car. They even managed to fly to Marseille together.

I was in France doing some *Rough Guide* work that summer and my cousins had lent us a house. Everyone – by that I mean the usual suspects: my mother, Jeremy's mother, the social worker – was convinced it was foolhardy and they were not up to it. I was anxious too, but I stuck to my belief that you have to let them try, to be independent, to live the kind of life they might have lived if illness had never struck them down. Thailand was one thing: the potential for calamity huge, but France? I was there, Jeremy is half French; he speaks French. That said, we both, Camilla and I, waited in utter trepidation for the arrival of their flight and when finally we caught sight of the two of them making their way through the last security barriers we burst into tears! Tears of relief, but also, for me, of joy and pride: that they had made it, that they had dared and done it.

We spent a week together. A difficult week, it has to be said. The girlfriend was docile and ready to fall in with other people's arrangements. Jeremy was volatile. He would be cheerful and relaxed and then suddenly lowering and hostile and you could never know why; there were no objective, observable reasons. Just the illness: those strange inward workings of the tortured mind, preoccupied by Lord-knows-what. I think he was happy, though, somewhere inside. We did not do much. It was difficult to get them interested in anything. We went to the lake and picnicked. They swam a little and lay on the bank smoking. Once or twice we managed to sit in a café, once we even ate, outside on the *terrasse* of course. Inside was too constraining for Jeremy: the uncomfortable proximity of strangers.

Contact, the rub, I said. This awful paranoia – what else to call it? – this fear of, hostility towards, anyone, everyone not known, that transforms a perfectly ordinary encounter over a shop counter, a brushing past in the street, a request for verification of your address when presenting a prescription at the chemist, into a situation fraught with fear and suspicion and potential for violence and aggression. It is the great curse of the illness for Jeremy, and for others, not all: it prevents you accepting the help and kindness that people offer in all sincerity, it makes friendship well-nigh impossible: it shuts you into a horrid, probably frightening, and lonely cocoon of isolation.

I do not remember how long the contact with *Umbrella*, the support group, lasted. Not long. It was a pity, because they were prepared to be very helpful if Jeremy had been willing to co-operate. But he took against them. The workers they sent round were probably young, not very experienced: they were this, they were that, couched always in pretty aggressive language, and he was not going to have anything more to do with them. The CPN had taken his back seat. Jeremy did not like the social worker. After a month or two, who knew what was going on but his mother and I?

And there were problems with his prescriptions. He was taking his medication in pill form and had to go to the GP to renew the prescriptions. That meant actually getting to the GP, going at particular times, often being asked to wait: all things which cause no difficulties for people who are well, but for someone in Jeremy's condition can become insuperable difficulties, obstacles weighted with inexplicable and indescribable problems. Yesterday, for example – to jump a few years in chronology: he went to the chemist for a prescription and the young girls who served him queried him, about his address, about his claim that he does not need to pay; why does not he need to pay?

'They were stupid girls, half my age,' he told me. 'I could have been their father. Why should I have to explain to them?' He lost his temper and was rude and left, without his medication.

An hour or so later I went round to find out what had happened. First, I saw that the girls at the counter were young Muslims with their heads wrapped in veils. I asked to speak to their manager. I had to wait several minutes. I positioned myself half way to the entrance to the chemist's back room to indicate that I was getting impatient. Eventually the manager/chemist came out. She was an intelligent, well-spoken and beautiful Pakistani girl. She was gentle and polite and explained that her employees were frightened and had only asked my son the questions they asked everybody. I suggested that in view of the nature of the medication requested on the prescription they should have been aware that they were dealing with someone with mental health problems and could have been a bit more sensitive.

She would not accept that there was any fault on their side. And perhaps in a way there was not. But cultural sensitivity? I am sick of hearing about it: just maybe, some day, someone might think about trying to show a little cultural sensitivity towards schizophrenics for a change. Or, provide some other means of getting their medication.

Who is to blame? Schizophrenia makes people behave strangely. Frequently they refuse to do the things that are clearly in their best interests and equally frequently they are unable, not because they are ill-mannered, uncouth or badly educated, to do perfectly normal, routine things in a normal, routine way, because of their condition. You find yourself saying, "Surely: one would have thought..." But these responses are simply wrong. We are running into the familiar cul-de-sac: we are not dealing here in the realm of reason.

But, one says nonetheless, doctors, chemists, surely ought to have some provision for dealing with such awkward and vulnerable customers. Is it beyond the wit of doctors to devise some system in their practices that highlights dangerously vulnerable patients and alerts them when these patients' prescriptions are due for renewal? Could they not try to make things easy for them? Could they perhaps devise some system for actually physically delivering the prescription to the patient?

The absence of such provision can be dangerous, as I was to learn most painfully.

It is not that Jeremy has never been able to establish a reasonably successful relationship with anybody; he has done so with some people, with some of his consultants, for example, the occasional social worker, one of his uncles. What accounts for this? What is it that enables some people to establish successful contacts with people like Jeremy?

I grew up with animals: dogs, horses, cattle, various animals at different times. We were always told not to be afraid or not to show fear in the presence of an animal, because animals sense fear, anxiety, uncertainty and that unsettles them. They "smell" confidence and benign intentions in humans and respond accordingly. I am sure something similar happens in human relations. The confidence or serenity that comes with feeling at home in your own skin, we sense that, or the absence of it, in each other, and the genuineness of feeling that accompanies it. Professional care or professed interest or care is something different. A normal, rational person can accept that, the practical help that a trained professional can provide; the question of the authenticity of the feelings of the person providing the help is not really relevant; it is a separate issue and unimportant. But for someone whose ability to make rational, objective assessments has, through illness, been destroyed and replaced by a generalised suspicion vis-à-vis the world, that "sense" of the other person becomes all-important.

I was travelling home by train from Birmingham one day in the 1990's when I was surprised to find a little boy, aged about five and apparently belonging to the woman sitting across the aisle, sniffing like a dog up and down the length of my arm which was resting on the aisle-side arm-rest. Seeing what was happening the woman apologised to me and explained that the boy was Romanian, rescued by her sister from an orphanage where he had been confined all his life with so little care and attention from anyone that he had not yet learnt to speak. Like an animal he had to rely on other senses to give him the information he needed about people.

When Jeremy has responded favourably to any of the professionals who have come his way, they have nearly always been people sufficiently confident in themselves to appear rather eccentric. One such was a community psychiatrist to whose care he was assigned after his first consultant retired. He came to work on a battered old-fashioned-looking motorbike. Often he kept his scuffed biker's boots on in his office. For Jeremy he obviously gave out the right vibe, for Jeremy continued to see him and ring him up for the five years until he too retired and Jeremy himself had long since slipped off the radar of any representative of the social services – not that they appeared to try very hard to maintain contact with such a recalcitrant patient. There were not enough of them to go round in the first place; I think it was probably quite welcome when a difficult patient either said he did not want to see them any more or missed so many appointments they had an excuse for taking him off the books.

*

People, friends, often ask me, "What does he do all day?" He does not go to work. He does not see friends very much, as he does not have many. He does not go to Day Centres. "I don't want to spend my time with nutters," he says. And it is true: they do seem to be rather dreary places, their habitués the same people you spend your time with when you are in a hospital psychiatric ward.

He stays at home. He reads, writes neat and sometimes abusive letters by the dozen, which he leaves, sealed in neatly stamped and addressed envelopes all over his flat, without ever posting them. He fills pages of notebooks with his writings, sometimes interesting and funny, sometimes strange and crazy. He sits and smokes and stares. He often has the radio or the telly on but with the sound, even on the radio, turned down so low that he cannot hear what is being said. Are they a substitute for company or do they help keep the torment of voices at bay? He makes a lot of phone calls, sometimes dozens, especially to his sister, and, when he is not well, leaves dozens of rude or crazy messages, which are unpleasant to receive, even when you know they are too mad to mean anything. Or there are periods when he comes to visit frequently, every day, sometimes two or three times. Then, suddenly, he will take himself off across the city to the Buddhist Society. I do not know what prompts this boldness, for generally he is too timid to use public transport to go very far. How long he stays when he gets there is hard to know. Sometimes, I get the impression, he leaves almost as soon as he has arrived. I do not know what they think of him. Sometimes I get the impression that they are not as understanding as you might expect such an organisation to be.

Isolation is the bane of the mentally ill. I do not know how he copes with such loneliness. I know he sometimes feels horribly alone. Yet I have also come to think that in some strange way the self-absorption, the preoccupation, the turned-inwardness that the illness seems to induce also, perhaps mercifully, protects the sufferer from what to the outside observer appears the extreme ghastliness of his condition.

*

It was around this time, when the first consultant retired and Jeremy was transferred to the Community Mental Health team, based in a day hospital only a few hundred metres from where he lived, that his medication was also changed, under pressure from me. Through the NSF we had been campaigning for several years by this time for patients to be prescribed drugs from the newer generation of anti-psychotic medication. They were said to target patients' symptoms more accurately rather than merely sedating their brain activity generally; in particular they targeted what are called the negative symptoms of schizophrenia, the tendency to paranoia, depression, lack of motivation, as well as causing fewer side effects like the notorious dyskinesia or involuntary shaking or twitching of hands or legs. Jeremy was given a drug called Risperidone and responded well to it. I think he did feel freer and less oppressed by it than his previous medication, but it too had to be taken orally and, like all medication, had to be taken absolutely religiously in order to achieve a therapeutic dose. He never refused it but he would miss a day or two, perhaps more sometimes; it was hard to know.

He continued to hear voices. Always they were associated with complaints about neighbours. He could hear the neighbours; they were bugging him. It was never really clear which neighbours. Sometimes he complained about the flats with whom he shared access to the courtyard and had to pass on the way to his own front door. Once or twice the occupants complained to me about him, in particular a young woman who turned out to be training as a social worker with mental health patients and was quite sympathetic. She was attractive and he had tried to talk to her, to chat her up, probably at times when she did not want to be disturbed. She had sliding glass doors along the courtyard side of her flat so that you could see in as you passed. Illness does not lessen your desire to strike up relationships with pretty women. She felt vulnerable and threatened.

Some other neighbours had a brick tossed through their window. They were an older couple and luckily were kind and understanding. Again I think the trouble arose because Jeremy had tried to be friendly and then felt rebuffed when he rang their doorbell, something he was quite likely to do at inappropriate times like seven in the morning, and they had asked him not to.

For this too is another peculiar consequence of the illness: a loss of the sense of what is appropriate. Impelled by imperatives you cannot control you do things, say things, in the urgency of the moment without the circumspection and calculation that is part of ordinary people's decision-making procedures.

Neighbours seem to serve, in a way I have never quite been able to understand, as the embodiment, the objectification of things going on in his own head. When he tries to explain the experience of hearing voices to me, it seems paradoxically that it is often a known, familiar voice that he hears and can clearly identify as, for example, his own sister's, yet which is associated with, even somehow embodied by, the neighbour. I say to him, 'If you can really hear the neighbours, put some music on or the radio, something to provide a screening noise of your own,' but of course if it is a projection of something going on in your own head that you are attributing to the neighbours, this is not very useful advice. This hearing of voices is such a central feature of schizophrenia and of Jeremy's own experience of it that I would like to be able to understand what exactly it feels like, what exactly he hears. Is it actual words? Conversations that could be repeated? Is it just noise, like snow on a television screen?

*

Much is made in official circles of the role of carers: how numerous we are, how important; how we have needs and rights, including the right to have our needs assessed: can we afford the bus fare to visit our "sufferer" in hospital or attend meetings to discuss our rights? If you follow any of this up, however, you quickly discover that applying for financial assistance under a carer's assessment automatically entails a reduction in the amount of disability living allowance your "sufferer" or "service user" receives! As soon as I discovered that I gave up trying to claim any allowances for myself. It is of course quite a costly business trying to ensure that someone whose only income is social security benefits enjoys a reasonable standard of living.

The London Borough of Camden organised carers' groups, the Royal Free Hospital also. During these years I started attending some of these meetings, partly because various mental health staff I was in touch with asked me to and partly out of a desire to relieve my own frustrations by deceiving myself into thinking I was doing something positive to advance the cause.

One of the things you quickly notice if you go to these meetings is that nobody else does. What is the figure? Eight million, I think. Eight million carers. They tell us how important we are, how dependent the health of the nation is upon the work we do, yet nobody goes to the meetings. Might not this just be evidence that whatever help the system thinks it is providing it is not the right help?

One of the Royal Free groups was helpful and relatively well attended; it was run by a psychologist for parents and family of people with schizophrenia. It was welcoming and supportive, in the same sort of way as my local NSF group; people went to talk about their specific problems and offer each other advice and sympathy. That of course was the group that was closed: on the grounds that it was duplicating work done elsewhere, although I never discovered where.

Another group I attended was run by Royal Free staff – bureaucrats – but at least mostly with a mental health background and thus some insider knowledge of the problems we faced. Speakers were invited, usually to tell us about plans and schemes in their various professional pipelines. Some talks were informative, about the effectiveness of different drugs, about supervised discharge from hospital, the role of key-workers and GPs: things that were of some practical use to us. But the moment the managerial people were involved, the bureaucrats from organisations like the Mental Health Commission, the emphasis shifted to what are now known as "issues around mental health": accommodating ethnic diversity, the provision of special diets and prayer facilities, obsessive concerns about confidentiality and patients' rights or, to my mind, footling transparency-accountability-customer-service issues. At one meeting, for instance, the hospital Service Development Manager – the title says it all – announced that in the hospital's main concourse there was now a "how we are doing board" and she proposed that a good subject for it would be this particular group because it was attended by carers, patients, professionals and "others that have dealings with our service", in other words, ticked the boxes and looked good. To that end, a photographer would be coming round. Of course anyone objecting to being photographed would be free to leave. God preserve us from violation of our human right to privacy, anonymity, non-participation... I left!

I used to find it difficult to keep my cool in these circumstances. One would have thought – wouldn't one? – that the main issue preoccupying all those attending meetings designed to serve the interests of people suffering from schizophrenia would be that illness, schizophrenia, and what could be done to alleviate it and improve the provision of treatment and care. Is it a matter even of tertiary importance and even to Albanians that cold tripe soup should be on the breakfast menu?

Much, of course, is also made of the importance of consultation, or at least of the appearance of consultation. But just as the current universality of customer service departments is a sure sign that the very last thing on the mind of the company concerned is service to its customers, so you can be pretty sure that those who seek to reassure you that no action will be initiated without full consultation have no serious intention of modifying the plans they have already made.

I remember two talks in particular. One was by a representative of the accountancy firm, Touche Ross. Their spokeswoman addressed us in business-speak; she talked about developing a business case for mental health services. I admit I know nothing of such matters, but the general impression given that in some sense the most important aspects of providing care for the mentally ill had to do with cost-cutting and purchasing and even, it seemed, in some peculiar way with showing some kind of profit, I found deeply disturbing and distasteful.

The other resulted in an acrimonious spat with the Mental Health Commissioner for Camden and Islington Health Authority and her bureaucrats. She came to talk to us about the Authority's commissioning intentions for 1996/97, but her talk was so obviously unprepared and so confused I had really no idea what she had been trying to tell us. And I said so.

I had walked out of a couple of other meetings and must have written a letter, which I no longer have a copy of. In front of me I have a reply signed on her behalf but written by her Commissioning Manager, dated February 7th 1996.

'I was concerned,' he writes, 'to discover your views about the consultancy exercise on acute services. Had you felt able to stay at the meeting held on January 10th 1996 where users' and carers' views on acute services were sought, you would have seen that the discussion was wide-ranging.' He ended his letter: 'Since I have twice addressed meetings that you have left in a degree of frustration, perhaps you would like to meet with me on a one-to-one basis. This might help you to understand the Health Authority's stance. For my part, I would not wish you to believe that I am unsympathetic to the carers of those people with mental illnesses. This is far from the truth.'

I replied on March 5th:

'Yes, I have indeed found attending your meetings a frustrating experience. At the Royal Free, I came to hear you tell us what provisions the Health Authority was making for the mentally ill in 1996. But you conducted the meeting in a manner so vague and rambling – unprepared, it seemed – that after an hour I still had no idea what you were trying to say, and I was not alone in that.

'Then, to compound the impression of woolliness, you sent me, after the January 10th meeting at St James' House, a letter which included the following paragraph: "I would be grateful if you have any comments, that they are fed back to me by 1st February 1996. Could I apologise for this short timescale, however the reason why we will need your comments is this tight schedule which we are working within to meet deadlines around these developments."

'A mangling of grammar, syntax and vocabulary, that hardly inspires confidence in the clarity or rigour of the thinking. And is not the word the thought?

'I fear it is. And that is another reason I have little confidence in your office. My impression is that you – and by "you" I mean the so-called professionals – are happier trading the shibboleths of the day among yourselves – that peculiar jargon of "empowering clients", "accessing services" and so on – than you are listening to the people, like parents, who have to live with the bizarre and often frightening reality of severe mental illness like schizophrenia every day.

'The current jargon – empowering, accessing, service-users, delivering services, service-providers, advocacy, client – implies a number of assumptions that, in my view, are inimical to the cause of the mentally ill. First, it implies a relation between the sick person and his healer that resembles that between the purchaser of a pound of peas and the shopkeeper more than that between what we used to call the patient and his doctor. Second, it seems to imply a sort of hostile intent on the part of the healer (at least, the prevalence of such terms as advocacy do): that treatment, whether clinical or other, is a sort of coercive intervention from which the "client" needs to be protected. Third, it implies that the sick person is a rational being capable of taking informed decisions about his own condition and treatment.

'When, at one of your meetings, I suggested that the jargon acted as a smokescreen preventing you from seeing the reality of life with schizophrenia and that there were often phases in the life of someone with schizophrenia when he, quite literally, was not "in his right mind", my remarks were greeted with a storm of protest. A representative of some advocacy or civil liberties outfit accused me of being patronising. Someone from Survivors Speak Out – the very name of that organisation speaks volumes – said he was offended and insulted and one of the professionals said I spoke from a "carer's point of view".

'My feeling is that your deliberations amount to little more than fiddling while Rome burns. Why don't you talk to the parents of people suffering from schizophrenia, with people, for example, who are members of the National Schizophrenia Fellowship or SANE? It is precisely the carers who know the reality.

'How often do people have a terrible time even getting their sick children admitted to hospital? Getting GPs or even so-called crisis-intervention teams to recognise that drastic help is required? What information are they given when hospital admission and diagnosis are finally achieved? Does anyone explain the likely prognosis? Offer advice about how best to deal with the illness? Explain what treatments are available? Explain the Care Programme Approach? Tell you about Care Plans – never mind putting them into effect? Explain the problems of housing or the possibility of sheltered housing? And how much sheltered accommodation exists? What happens if there is no place available? What happens if your child lives on his own? Who is going to keep an eye on him? And, if he won't let them in, who is going to know how he is and how quickly will they find out, before something goes seriously wrong? And many other questions that you could not provide a satisfactory answer to.

'I suppose you must be aware of it: the support system for schizophrenics not in hospital is woefully inadequate, full of potentially lethal holes. The most fundamental provisions for their care have simply not been made. They have a right to be treated in a civilised society. They are not easy to treat, we know that, for their illness interferes with the normal processes of thinking. But tiptoeing around uncomfortable truth, talking of empowerment and so forth, is not any help to anybody.'

I received a very prompt reply.

'I apologise for the poor grammar to which you drew my attention. I was not the author of the letter concerned and am therefore not responsible for the thought content [he had signed it!]... I am sorry that you found the meeting at the Royal Free unhelpful. It is very difficult in a mixed group of professionals, carers and users to know at what level to pitch a presentation... I will not engage in the other points in your letter. You clearly have a very fixed view, to which you are entitled. However, there are many widely differing views around mental health services and mental ill health. I think you should know that I have worked in the mental health field for many years and have had close contact with users of services and their carers over those years.'

And why, one wants to ask, are there so "many widely differing views around mental health services and mental ill health" and not, say, "around" heart or kidney disease or cancer? And why is it that so many amateurs – by which I mean people without much scientific medical training: social workers, for example, not to mention mental health bureaucrats – feel entitled to hold views about mental illness when they would be very shy of holding forth about the most appropriate treatments for heart disease?

It is now the year 2008: twelve years have elapsed and still the questions I asked in the penultimate paragraph of my letter quoted above could be put with just the same urgency. And, to make matters worse, today the authorities – now known as the Camden and Islington NHS Foundation Trust – are cutting services in order to save money while dressing the exercise up as streamlining, rationalising, modernising, accommodating women's issues, issues of cultural diversity... Their response to my kind of objection, just the same.

When they can, the bureaucrats always claim a long history of involvement in mental health. But I am not much impressed by the quality – intellectual, in particular – of the people who work "in the field of mental health". I am not referring to medical staff: they have had to undergo a rigorous education. It is the other services that I have my doubts about. First of all, mental health is a pretty unglamorous, unrewarding and difficult area to work in. There is a very high proportion of black immigrants with poor language skills – that is to say, they cannot speak English intelligibly – employed among the lower echelons. This is not because blacks are especially gifted at or particularly attracted to the caring professions; it is because these are jobs that better qualified people do not want and, being in the public sector, have at the same time a certain cachet of respectability, especially for people who come from cultures where being a public employee and wearing the uniform of the state gives a certain status and power. There are certainly some saintly people among them, people with real compassion, but when they move, generally for career reasons, into management and administration their shortcomings are quickly shown up. Secondly, I have never seen any reason to be any more impressed by the quality of the bureaucrats, the people who man the administration of these services, still largely white. It would be interesting to know how many of them have a social work or similar background, from which a side-step into administration – rather as with teachers escaping from the classroom – might seem an escape into relative peace and quiet. Besides, who, one wants to ask, with any ambition or real get-up-and-go would choose a career in hospital administration?

How can you have any faith in the proposals of people who apparently do not notice that there is anything odd in saying things like: "More services from non-statutary (*sic*) agencies such as therapies moving across service provision therefore enabling a greater choice and services tailored to individual needs" or "In doing this work we should now draw a line under thinking about Friern reprovision and look at needs in their entirety including the next generation of people requiring this level of care"?

Chapter Seven
Some Calm Before A Storm

In 1997 my parents died, my father in January, my distraught mother six months later. Jeremy bravely came to both funerals and in spite of the presence of many people he did not know coped pretty well. The presence of his numerous cousins helped. They are loyal, loving and accepting, although they are much younger and do not know him well. Feeling them all about him, and his uncles too, feeling part of a clan was and remains a big support for him.

At my father's funeral he sat with me and his much loved granny. He was terribly upset by her grief. Afterwards, at the wake, he put in an occasional appearance, withdrawing from time to time to what had been his room as a child, where he sat quietly smoking.

At night, having said goodnight to Mum who insisted on sleeping as usual in the bed in which Dad had so recently died – poor thing: I think she was just dazed by animal grief, her husband of nearly sixty years torn from her so suddenly, a husband whom she had railed against often enough but upon whose utter dependence on her she herself had finally become dependent – I went in to see Jeremy. His room was opposite Mum's. His light was on. He was asleep, lying on his side, under the covers but with his clothes on. On the bedside table lay an ashtray full of the brown, chewy remains of roll-ups. In the bookcase were books we had read together when as a child he came to stay with his grandparents. There was a model we had made of Speke Hall in Cheshire, a kestrel we had found dead in Camden Town that I had had stuffed and mounted in a glass-fronted cabinet that I had made for him and painted with what I imagined was an appropriate sort of background landscape in watercolour. For a while I watched him sleeping, peacefully, in his childhood bed surrounded by these mementoes of happier times when divorce and separation and illness and death had not even been shadows on anyone's horizon. If only it had been ever thus, if only we could turn back the clock...

I do not know about humankind not being able to bear too much reality, but I do know that the sadness of it is sometimes unbearable.

I was up a ladder cleaning windows when Mum had phoned to tell me she was terribly worried about Dad. 'I'll come right away,' I told her, but he died before I could get there to say goodbye. And I never managed to say goodbye to her either.

After Dad died we decided, with my brothers, that we would make sure that Mum never spent a night alone. Camilla and I drove up every weekend and the others took care of the weekdays or arranged for some friend to sleep in. We managed never to leave her alone until, early one morning in June, my second brother phoned to say that the friend sleeping over had found Mum dead at six that morning.

The friend was a down-to-earth farmer's wife. It took me a year to pluck up the courage to phone and thank her for being there on Mum's last night of life. When I did so, I could not speak for sobbing. She said, 'It's a terrible thing for a boy to lose his mother.' I was fifty-five.

She was right. I felt very alone and exposed, as if, so to speak, my base area had been overrun: there was no longer a last line of defence to withdraw to, nowhere to fall back. Without Camilla, I would have been frightened.

In August we took Jeremy and his girlfriend to Ireland for a week to stay in our family house. We had a pint or two at our local, sitting outside looking over the sea. We went for a walk or two along the beach. Many cigarettes were smoked. We did not do very much, for as usual they did not want to do very much. Probably there was a fair bit of moroseness and tension, but photographs show that there were happy moments too.

On our last day Princess Diana died. We were tidying up, preparing to leave, when Tae announced that she had just heard on the radio about the fatal car accident. I do not remember the exact sequence of events. Jeremy shouted angrily at Camilla for being rude to Tae and told her to fuck off. I told him no one had been rude to anyone. 'We have had a really nice week together. Let's not spoil it now.' He told me to fuck off and when I remonstrated with him he went for me, caught me with a blow to my cheek and another to my mouth so rapidly I was unable to defend myself. I seized a chair to hold him off. He was pale with fury, beside himself.

There was a terrible silence. I went to examine the damage in a mirror and find a piece of tissue to staunch the bleeding. I said, 'Jeremy, what are you doing? I'm your father. You could have really hurt me.'

My face was running with blood. Tae looked shocked. We were all shocked, including Jeremy. We got in the car and drove off. I stopped in Oughterard to show my face to the chemist. She said she thought I probably ought to have a stitch but could not do it herself. I said I had to go to London, so she gave me something to staunch the bleeding and hold the edges of the wound together.

Somewhere in the first half hour, in a quiet and frightened voice, barely audible, Jeremy apologised. Apart from that hardly a word was spoken during the thirty-six hours it took us to get back to London.

And life returned to normal. Jeremy lay low for several days. He was terribly contrite, as he always is after a row; I think he had frightened himself as well. Whenever we talk of going to Ireland or even of going away anywhere together now – and eleven years have elapsed – he says he is frightened of what happened then, although he has never been violent with me since.

In September he went into hospital for a fortnight's respite because of "mental health deterioration: paranoid ideation and auditory hallucination", as the official document puts it. Today I do not think going into hospital as a "respite" measure would be possible, because of the reduction in the number of in-patient beds made for reasons of economy.

Restored, he returned to his flat and thus began a period of four years of relative calm, that is to say, a period in which nothing drastically untoward happened: no hospital admissions, no dramatic relapses. A period of routine anxiety for me: anxious bike rides over to Kilburn in response to appeals to "come and see me". Cleaning sessions, unblocking drains. I had to maintain the entrance courtyard too, as none of the other residents ever bothered to repair or paint the door, replace light bulbs or weed the unkempt flowerbed.

Jeremy muddled along. Happy and not happy, his moods volatile and changeable. Tae was still part of his life for the first two or three years. I never quite understood how their relationship worked. She had moved house with her mother and her mother had forbidden her to give Jeremy either the address or telephone number, so the poor chap had to wait, in helpless dependence, for Tae to phone, for Tae to decide whether or not she was coming over. When she complained to me about Jeremy being difficult, I told her off: I said it was most unfair to expect to continue the relationship and yet not even give him a telephone number.

The elderly Czechs, the freeholders of Jeremy's building, whose business occupied the two lower floors, left and were replaced by a strange unkempt fellow who looked like a tramp. He moved in and lived on the premises. I was worried that this might lead to conflicts. Jeremy did occasionally complain that he could hear someone playing the guitar or that the radio was on late, but there was no trouble. Perhaps their different strangenesses cancelled each other out. Another neighbour complained to me that Jeremy was peeing out of one of the windows overlooking the shared courtyard. I thought this most unlike him and, given the configuration of his flat, a singularly inconvenient way of relieving himself. I asked which window and was shown a window which belonged to the apartment of the new tramp-like freeholder.

Jeremy did look odd. He did behave strangely. He was unpredictable. He was sometimes offensive and aggressive. But did that mean he was also likely to pee out of windows? Once a nutter, I suppose, always a nutter. Some people coped with this strangeness better than others. Right outside the communal front door lived a couple who were wonderfully understanding. The husband was the one who saw most of Jeremy, for he worked on the street, repairing cars. He was always cheerful and friendly. If

Jeremy did not respond he paid no attention. If Jeremy wanted to stop and chat, he chatted. He took no offence.

There were the inevitable complaints from Jeremy about the neighbours when he was not well, their voices and noise, but there were no actual confrontations. He took his pills and did not take his pills. It was hard to know with what regularity he took them or missed them. There were always those little silvery plaquettes lying about with some pills still nesting in their places, untouched. Clearly he took them most of the time, as he always assured me. How much better might he have been had he taken them scrupulously?

There were periods when he almost flourished. He took himself off on a week-long residential Buddhist retreat once. How much he was actually able to participate, I do not know, but he got himself there and back. There were times when Tae seemed almost to have moved in with him. There were a couple of scares about pregnancy: scares for Tae at least, because she was frightened of her mother, and for me, because I was terrified of what the consequences might be. Jeremy always talked about having babies and indeed still does; he would have loved to have children.

Although Tae always looked neat and clean and fresh herself, her presence made not the slightest difference to the state of the flat. What would they have done with children? How could they have fed, clothed and cared for them? Any child would have been taken into care immediately.

I tried hard when I went round to restrain my desire to clear up, wash up, empty the bath or offer advice about how to live better. He did not like it and often said so. "Sit down, Dad, and let me see you. I don't like it when you come round and starting acting like a servant." It must have seemed like an implicit criticism, that whatever he did was not enough. He did make some effort to tidy up. There was often laundry hung up to dry. And the fact is, the place never seized up altogether.

What did we do? We played backgammon, occasionally chess. I asked him about Buddhism. He told me about his writing.

I loved him and wanted to help and make things better. Yet it was so hard, even really to have an ordinary conversation: he had no ordinary life, poor boy, no friends, no regular occupation, no exchange, no interaction with anybody, just the brief daily excursions to the shop round the corner to buy cigarettes, milk, the few odds and ends of things that he drank and ate. And even a visit to the familiar shop was too much sometimes; he would be back within a few minutes, having been unable to face the street or, perhaps, pass a particular person. Only two or three friends from the old days kept in some sort of touch. One, a friend from school days, was busy being married and raising a family, but has always – and still is – kind and understanding enough to be there at the end of the phone when, sometimes after long intervals, Jeremy decides to contact him. Another, a friend from university days, travels the world as a teacher but has never lost touch. I feel deeply grateful to them. A couple of others hover on the fringes of his life, both, I think, with troubles of their own.

And all this time he received no help from anyone. There was no social worker, no CPN, no care co-ordinator. His contact with the system that was supposed to be taking care of him was Dr C. I don't know how often he phoned or how often he saw him but he did at least maintain the contact. For a time we had regular meetings – Care Plan meetings, I suppose they were – but then they ceased too; I think it was because Jeremy had said he did not want to go on having such meetings or did not want his parents to be involved. So, in effect, no one apart from his mother and father, no one official had any idea for a couple of years about the state of health of this person with a potentially dangerous illness.

To compound things, Dr C retired and Tae, after various alarms and threats, finally ended her relationship with Jeremy, leaving him terribly unhappy and even more alone. There was nothing he could do; he could not phone her because he did not have her number. He tried to find her by searching the streets in the area where he knew she lived. For years he waited every Sunday at the church she attended with her mother on the off chance of being able to speak to her.

In 2001 I set off to walk across France. I was gone for three months. Every day, as I emerged from woods, crossed fields on to country lanes, entered village squares, I 'kept fourteen eyes', as the Greeks say, on the lookout for public phones. Mostly they were in working order, unlike English ones, although the remotest had an inconvenient habit of wanting coins rather than cards, which kept our conversations short. Sometimes he would say he missed me and keep asking when I would be back. Other times he seemed to be coping well enough. Occasionally I would check with his mother but I tried to avoid that as she always gave such a pessimistic and gloomy account of the situation: I would be depressed and anxious for two or three days afterwards.

I returned home towards the end of July. I remember going to see Jeremy the day after I got back. Sunlight was pouring cheerfully into his living-room. He did not look particularly unwell, but there was a degree of disorder in the flat that spoke of madness, not just a normal untidiness. He assured me he was okay. Then for two or three days he would not speak to me, did not answer the phone: a familiar enough response, a kind of punishment he reserves for me when I have been away.

It was a Sunday when he phoned again. His voices were troubling him and he was obviously rather frightened. I asked if he had taken his pills and he confessed that he had not had any medication for more than three weeks. He did not even have any in the house; he had been too frightened to walk the ten minutes or so to the surgery to pick up a new prescription. I said I would come over and we would find the duty chemist for that Sunday.

We duly found him. We were perhaps half a mile from Jeremy's flat. As we were driving back he said he could hear his neighbour. He called him a bastard, I think. He always swore about the people whose voices he "heard". I tried to reassure him that it could not be the neighbour in any literal sense; physically it just was not possible to hear him at this distance.

'Why don't you come home with me?' I said, but he did not want to.

I left him at his flat. We spoke on the phone later in the day. He seemed fine. On Monday morning he phoned me again, sounding much better, even cheerful. We said we would meet later. Little did I know that this would turn out to be one of the most frightening days of my life.

At about four in the afternoon the phone rang. I expected it to be Jeremy, but it was the neighbour we did not like, the one who had accused Jeremy of pee-ing out of the window, the one whose voice he had complained of hearing in the car. He told me that Jeremy had just been taken away by the police and was on his way to hospital. He said Jeremy had rung his doorbell and threatened him. He was not hurt but had called the police.

My worst nightmare realised at last: my son, my child, locked up for ever in a secure hospital-prison. How could such a thing have happened? Thank God Mum had not lived to see such a thing. What to do? I did not know what to do. There was no point in going round to the flat now that Jeremy had gone. I could not think what to do. Anguish was what I felt: my whole body felt flayed. Camilla volunteered to come with me and together we walked up to the hospital; I assumed he would be taken to the Royal Free.

In fact he had arrived shortly before us. He was in a cell-like room with a big window through which he could be kept under surveillance. He was being minded by a shaven-skulled Neanderthal thug in a suit that was too tight for his shoulders, the sort of muddy-brained goon it has become fashionable to have guarding pubs and clubs. There were two or three police officers in uniform. There was a good deal of to-ing and fro-ing. We were in some area of the Accident and Emergency department, I think. I do not know how I got there, how I found him; I do not remember asking, I do not remember who told me where to go to find someone brought in by the police. There was a sort of reception desk, some nurses and at least one doctor, a psychiatrist, to whom I was introduced. He had an obviously Greek name, I noted.

I asked if I could talk to Jeremy and he immediately let me into the holding room and, when I hesitated, asked the goon to leave. Jeremy was terribly pale and looked bewildered. I embraced him, briefly, as we were in full public view; I wanted to cry. I said something like, 'It's okay, love. It will be all right.' I asked him what had happened. He said the neighbour had been bugging him, so he wanted to give him a fright. He had not intended to hurt him, just frighten him. The neighbour claimed Jeremy had come after him. Who knows exactly what happened?

He had gone back into his flat, he said, after the incident and then the police had arrived, with plastic shields, banging on the door and shouting to him to come out with his hands on his head and he had been handcuffed.

I talked to the police officer who seemed to be in charge. He was extraordinarily nice and sympathetic. He too, it turned out, had a Greek connection; he used to go sailing there. He tried to reassure me. I wanted to know what the possible outcome of an episode like this might be. He said the neighbour could press charges and there would have to be an assessment by a forensic psychiatrist and that this was not necessarily a bad thing because it would mean that Jeremy would be kept in hospital and properly supervised.

Eventually the police left. Jeremy wanted to go for a pee and had to be accompanied by the goon, who did not quite frog-march him, but close... a precaution I thought rather unnecessary. The goon was, I assumed, the employee of some private security contractor, not NHS staff. (How can you expect appropriate behaviour in the age of sub-contracting? What training has a goon like this had for dealing with disturbed psychiatric patients?)

I had by this time struck up a nicely complicit and friendly relationship with the Greek psychiatrist. I had said to him, in Greek, 'You must be Greek with a name like that.' So I was able to get information and advice without anyone else understanding what was being said. He explained that he could not have Jeremy admitted formally and found a bed in a ward until he had been visited by the duty social workers. These, he said, were two young women, aged about twenty-five. They had been sent for and would come down shortly to speak to Jeremy and ask him if he wanted to stay in hospital. If Jeremy said no, then he would have to release him. I said, surely, in view of what has happened, Jeremy had to be kept in hospital. 'You would think so,' the psychiatrist said, 'but this is the ridiculous system we have to work with.' 'What can we do?' I said. So together, in Greek, we concocted a plan to persuade these two girls that Jeremy was in real need of admission and to prevent them if possible from actually asking him the direct question.

In due course the social workers turned up. The psychiatrist used his Greek charm and we got them to accept his view that Jeremy should be admitted without the dangerous question ever being popped. Another hour or so and a bed was found for him on the old familiar ward. He was safe.

I kissed him goodbye and told him I would come round in the morning with some clothes and his washing things. Camilla and I walked home, with some feeling of relief. Things could have been worse. I was worried about the future, about the possible implications of prosecution, but at least there was no blood, no wounds, no injuries. I found it hard to believe that my son would actually have hurt a man, but you have to recognise that, with illnesses like this, it is literally possible to be "out of your mind", to be so impelled by forces beyond your control that you act in a manner quite out of character. Those who, out of attachment to a dogma no matter how idealistic or well-intentioned, find such a notion unpalatable are running a dangerous risk.

When we got home, I was exhausted. These are ghastly moments. That the destiny of your own child should have turned out so grim... I do not know how I would manage if it were not for Camilla. How could you face such bleakness alone? Yet people do. There are those in my group who do.

I went over to the flat in the dark, reluctant and full of a nameless emptiness. I wanted to make sure it was safe, everything locked.

Through the courtyard. Luckily the threatened neighbour was nowhere to be seen. The courtyard door was unlocked. Up the stairs. The flat door was locked. Into the flat. I put the lights on. Just the usual disorder: full ashtrays, empty and half-drunk beer cans, some laundry on the clothes-horse, dirty plates in the kitchen... I howled. It was a kind of death. All our effort to create niceness, warmth, comfort, beauty, cosiness, safety... Would this ever be home again?

But you have to act. A few wrenching sobs and a catharsis takes place sufficient to enable me to act. I gathered a few clothes from the wardrobe, some tobacco and papers, a book I knew he had been reading, locked everything securely and left. I did not go back for a week; I could not face it.

With Jeremy safe in hospital, we returned to the familiar routine. Neon days on Nicol Ward, nylon curtains the only privacy, rubbing shoulders with the poor, the crazed, the broken. But safe. And safer, because under "section" for six months. He grumbled about that at first, threatening to appeal, but I think secretly he was relieved too.

The threat of prosecution and problems with the police receded. The neighbour decided not to press charges. Regularly medicated once more, Jeremy returned to relative stability, neither really well, nor really unwell: better some days than others. He was allowed out on leave during the day, to buy tobacco, sit in cafés, visit his parents. There were the usual problems associated with hospital: conflicts with other patients, sometimes violent; lending money to others, sometimes clearly under duress, and not getting paid back; having his mobile phone stolen...

And then you begin to understand how difficult life can become when you do not fit the routine categories of the workaday world. The phone company will not deal with me because I am not the account holder. I have to explain to them – and of course they know nothing about schizophrenia – that their customer is in hospital suffering from an illness, which makes it difficult... And of course you do not want to give them too much information in case they refuse to insure anything ever again, possibly even to allow him a contract ever again. You have to describe the circumstances in which the phone was lost. Well, it was left on a hospital bed... He did not report it immediately. Nothing in our situation fits the assumptions made by insurance companies about the way events in the world are likely to unfold.

To do them justice, in the end – after numerous letters and explanations over the phone – they pay up. To avoid similar problems in the future I open the next account in my name: which of course means more bureaucratic preoccupations for me and a different set of complications when anything goes wrong. For example, when there is some kind of breakdown and Jeremy does not want me "interfering in" or "running his life", his phone remains out of order until he can be persuaded to let me get involved again. And so it is with gas bills and electricity bills and freedom passes: we are misfits, oddballs and there is a price to pay for non-conformity.

On Thursdays there are ward rounds, in effect a private meeting between the patient and his consultant psychiatrist and the "team" assigned to looking after him. Sometimes this can mean ten or twelve people, especially if there are students present. Average attendance is perhaps six or seven: subordinate doctors, nurses, occupational therapists, social workers, the people involved or to be involved in the daily supervision of the patient. Jeremy's mother and I would turn up at most meetings.

It is intimidating for the patient. He is summoned into the presence, a bit like a prisoner being led into the dock. The consultant asks how you are. If you are feeling pretty crazy and irrational the pretence at normal conversation that everybody feels obliged to maintain seems little more than a charade. I know that I would not have enjoyed being asked about "my voices" and other intimate matters in the presence of strangers.

Sometimes Jeremy performed with a good grace and sometimes he was angry and prickly; he might refuse to attend altogether or get up and leave, calling them all a bunch of wankers. The new consultant, a sympathetic, kindly woman, took it in good part. I went along because it reminded everyone that Jeremy's parents were an important part of his support system and that our views and role needed to be taken into consideration: a reminder that he was our son and that we had known him a lot longer and more intimately than any of the professionals, something which some of them, in their professional arrogance, have a tendency to forget, in spite of the theoretical/textbook emphasis on the importance of the carer. I also wanted everyone to know that I was on the case, prepared to make trouble if I thought things were not going right.

It is not the skill and judgement of the consultants that concern me. They are scientists, trained to look at evidence, identify facts and call them by their proper name. It is the so-called care services that I have always been and remain deeply sceptical of. Induction into these services is a) much less rigorous intellectually and b) conditioned by the ideology, the intellectual fashion of the day, not fact and analysis, but woolly-minded wishful thinking. The doctors call the people they treat patients: they see them as people suffering from problems whose origins can be traced and identified and then treated, within the limits imposed by the state of the medical art of the day. The social services see them as "clients", with all that implies. In a ward round meeting you will hear the subject of the meeting referred to as a patient by the doctors and a client by the support services, a difference which in my view points to a potentially dangerous divergence of approach.

Chapter Eight
Unsettled Times

Weeks and months go by. At first it is a relief to have Jeremy in hospital, even though visits are painful reminders of the depths to which he has sunk, the awful intractability of his illness and the undignified and humiliating conditions of the existence it has reduced him to. Then you start to worry about what the future may hold. He is better but he is not really well, not in the sense that he can go out into the world and manage by himself: food, cleanliness, bills, accommodation, getting around. He cannot go back to his flat. The threatened neighbour is still there; besides, even the nice, understanding neighbours down the street said that they and others would organise a campaign to prevent his return. That hurt. Am I the only person who can see the essential goodness in my son? Does he really seem that crazy, that dangerous and undesirable to the rest of the world?

I had let the flat. I could not afford to leave it empty. After Jeremy's admission to hospital, I had emptied everything, taking all his books, re-useable furniture and other effects to my brother's. It grieved me to do it; it was like clearing away my mother's things after she had died. I got Geoff to help me strip the whole place down, re-paint, lay new floors, make a new bathroom. I used to hate being there alone. When Geoff had to go back to his own work, I used to feel sick, with that hollow sinking feeling that I remembered from going back to school as a child. And then when it was all ready, looking better than it had ever done, I had to let a stranger move in, not my son. Would he ever be able to return to his own home?

No one believed he was ready to live on his own again, but equally he could not stay in hospital for ever. 2002 came and almost went. Housing is a matter for the Council. In December Jeremy's needs were assessed by the Housing Support Team who decided that the most appropriate solution would be what they call a supported housing scheme, in other words, a hostel. At a ward round in January 2003 the decision was taken to refer him to the same St Mungo's hostel where he had lived prior to moving into his own flat. The wheels of the bureaucracy began to turn, slowly, as usual. When I asked why it was taking so long, the hospital staff complained that they had issued repeated invitations to the Housing Officer to come to a ward round but no one ever came. In the meantime St Mungo's rejected Jeremy's referral. We were told that the Housing Team would appeal against the rejection, as there was still a vacancy there. Three weeks went by without any contact with the Housing Officer. Absolutely nothing was done. I wrote to the Housing Officer myself. It was the end of March. No reply. I wrote to St Mungo's, pleading with them to reconsider their decision, which had been taken on the grounds that they were not able to manage someone with Jeremy's "support needs" – politically correct, non-judgemental code for saying they were afraid he might be aggressive. By this time of course there were not any vacancies left.

I wrote to my MP, Glenda Jackson, whose intervention duly elicited a response from the Housing Support manager. As usual, any criticism is filed in the bureaucratic Council mind as a "complaint"; they appear to be categorically incapable of understanding that one might be offering a critique of the entire system. And of course there is a procedure for dealing with complaints, which is duly activated whenever one "complains". They investigate themselves: have all their procedures been duly followed? Invariably, they find that, yes, they have. And then they offer a little concession to the complainant:

'I do acknowledge that the process of coordination between all services involved in Mr S's care has not been of the highest quality, we would be (*sic*) addressing some of these issues by; a) ensuring regular face-to-face meetings with ward and mental health staff as well as Mr S to update on the progress of referrals and review any further action that may need to be taken. We expect that such meetings would take place every 2-3 weeks while we try to access suitable accommodation for Mr S; b) following up any referral to supported housing schemes on a 2-weekly basis and notify all interested parties of progress and any follow up action that may be need (*sic*) in writing.'

I had pointed out in my letter that there was an appalling lack of suitable accommodation available for people like my son. The Housing Support manager's letter went on:

'To address some of these issues, the team alongside other referral agencies and housing providers have already started some work looking at how we better coordinate assessments and referrals to reduce the duplication in services particularly with regards to managing referrals jointly to cut the waiting times for decisions and indeed the need for clients to have to go through more than one assessment process.

'Camden is also working with providers to create capacity within schemes by improving move on options for existing residents who may no longer need the services offered by supported housing providers.

'In the medium to long term, Camden Supporting People Team would be involved in the remodelling and commissioning of new supported housing services in the borough to meet the need of Camden residents.'

If pigs had wings...

This letter was written in July 2003. We went through all this confusion all over again in 2005 and 2006.

*

Towards the end of 2003 Jeremy reluctantly agreed to accept a place in a hostel run by *MIND*. There was not really any alternative, except the ghastly prospect of bed and breakfast in King's Cross.

I liked the hostel. The staff were sympathetic and committed. The manager, in spite of a discouraging appearance – every inch of visible skin tattooed or pierced, was kind and understanding, approachable, yet firm: exactly the kind of person needed in this sort of job. The building was an attractive Victorian house. The street was quiet. There was a villagey centre not far off, with cafés, a bookshop and some animation.

The house inevitably had that cold, impersonal, public air common to all such institutions, where nothing belongs to any individual. There was a communal sitting-room downstairs but nobody used it except a silent middle-aged man with long lank hair who always opened the door when you rang the bell. In fact, I don't think I ever saw another resident in the eighteen months Jeremy was there.

Jeremy's room was upstairs. It overlooked a garden, spacious but unkempt, because the hostel budget did not run to upkeep; if a room needed redecorating the staff had to do it. The room faced north, so was always filled with a rather discouraging, melancholy light. There was a bathroom and loo, shared with another resident, a woman, harmless but completely loopy. There was a sink in the room, a bed, a table, a wardrobe and a small chest of drawers: utility stuff, anonymous, characterless, used by countless others. What else would you expect?

You never saw anyone but heard in the distance the muffled bang of doors and footsteps on stairs.

There was a communal kitchen but Jeremy scarcely ever used it. Instead he ordered takeaways or bought a plastic sandwich from the petrol station at the corner of the street. So much for support, for needs being met: what more fundamental need is there than keeping body and soul together in a reasonably healthy manner by eating regular and balanced meals? And if he had not had a mobile phone he would have been in effect *incommunicado*. No one answered the communal hostel phone or if they did there was no guarantee they were going to go upstairs and find the person asked for.

Jeremy was not happy and he was not well. In fact, in spite of receiving his medication by fortnightly depot injection he was crazier than I had seen him in many a long year. It was depressing and distressing. Who was going to look after him? Who was going to take responsibility for making sure he was safe, for making him better? I wrote to the social worker, yet another, who of course had not made any effort to establish a relationship with me or Jeremy's mother. I wrote to the consultant, a man now, as it was thought Jeremy might respond better to a man. He acted.

They took Jeremy back into hospital for a couple of weeks and adjusted his medication. Then back to the hostel. Sometimes he was relatively well, sometimes not. We went for walks in the neighbouring playing fields. He would go and sit on a bench in the local cemetery and smoke. Sometimes we sat in the hostel garden. Sometimes we just sat in the car. He was lonely. For a while there was a surge of activity; one of his few remaining friends organised some trips into town at night. They went and looked at the girls and drank too much. I was pleased he could manage to do something "normal", go out on the town like any other young man, yet terrified they would get into trouble: that someone might pick on them for being strange and different. Miraculously there were no mishaps. But the party phase did not last very long. He got bored with the friend or the friend's friends. He pined for the lost Korean girlfriend and went every Sunday to see if he could speak to her at the church she attended.

The hostel manager left. There was not enough funding to sustain his post. The hostel had once been a registered care home, manned seven days a week, with a qualified nurse able to monitor residents' medication. Now there were staff only from Monday to Friday and no nurse among them, so no one was permitted to give out or in any way monitor medication. This, in a hostel with eight out of ten residents on Enhanced Care Programmes, that is to say, with a history of psychiatric illness sufficiently serious for them to be regarded as above averagely vulnerable.

Camden Council had decided to cut more than £60,000 from its Housing and Outreach services budget in the middle of the year, after its recipients had planned their expenditure for the year. The hostel staff told me this. I said I would write and object. I did, to Mr Ajibola Awogboro, the Mental Health Commissioner. I asked him what the policy on housing for the mentally ill was to be over the next few years and how they were going to reconcile making the improvements outlined in the Housing Support manager's letter to Glenda Jackson (see above) with cuts in the budget. I received no reply.

In December we learnt that the hostel would be completely unsupervised for several days over Christmas. The staff were themselves not happy about this arrangement. When I phoned to discuss the matter I found a locum, who told me he was shocked to discover that people on Enhanced Care Plans were going to be left for so long without any support over a period as notoriously difficult emotionally as Christmas. He also told me he thought it most inappropriate, indeed potentially dangerous, that when nearly all the residents were men the only staff should be young women. I see from a letter that I wrote to Glenda Jackson about this matter on December 15th 2004 that my son had been knocked down by another resident in a fight over some laundry on the previous day. What if this sort of thing should happen during a period when there were no staff about for several days?

I contacted our local newspaper, the *Hampstead and Highgate Express*, who put the story on the front page. After Christmas I found a message on my answer phone from Glenda Jackson. I called her back and she scolded me for going to the papers with the story. She said she had spoken to *MIND* and they had told her that it was their policy not to have staff in the hostel all the time because the residents were being empowered and enabled and prepared for moving on. I said, 'Well, they would say that. They were giving you the party line. All caring professions and charities talk like that nowadays. I have been involved with schizophrenia for nearly twenty years. I have talked to lots of people in the same boat. All this talk about empowerment is inappropriate for people suffering from schizophrenia. They are not going to move on. They need stability, security. They need supervision. They need someone to help them eat properly, keep clean, take their medication, get out of bed in the morning. Some manage better than others, but by and large you don't recover from schizophrenia and go back to work, back to normal life.' She said she too had talked to lots of people and accused me of wanting to go back to the bad old days of the lunatic asylum. She said she knew people who had been so disempowered by that experience that they had even forgotten how to use a light switch. I told her the hostel used to be a registered care home and almost certainly would be still if it were not for financial constraints. I told her the manager's post had been suppressed for reasons of economy. I said, 'If money were no object, there would be staff there at Christmas and at weekends too.'

As we were clearly at loggerheads, I said I did not think there was much point in continuing our conversation. As a final point I told her what the locum had said to me about the dangers of having only women staff at the hostel. 'That's gender bias,' she told me crossly. I said I thought it was plain common sense. And we ended our conversation there. I have to say that in spite of that spat she has continued to help me whenever I have turned to her.

MIND also complained about my going to the press.

About a week later my son phoned at ten o'clock in the evening. 'Will you come and get me, Dad? I'm scared.'

'What's the matter?'

'The fire brigade is here. That *** X has set fire to the office.'

X was the black man who before Christmas had hit him so hard he knocked him down. He lived on the floor below Jeremy. They had a history of conflict going back over various hospital admissions. One might have thought putting them in the same hostel was not the wisest thing to do.

I got in the car and drove up to the hostel. It was only a few minutes away. There were a couple of fire engines. Nothing seemed to be burning any more but firemen were still moving about in their fire-fighting gear looking like giants in the darkness. They asked me if I knew who they should contact. 'No,' I said, 'there are no staff at night or weekends.'

A couple of weeks later a member of staff told me *MIND* were threatening to evict Jeremy for shouting at and being aggressive towards another resident. They had convened a meeting with the social worker, key worker and *MIND* housing manager, which Jeremy had been summoned to attend. I wrote to *MIND*, to the social worker (yet another one who had not bothered to make contact either with me or Jeremy's mother) and to the consultant.

To the social worker I wrote (Feb 2nd 2005):

'I am Jeremy's father. I am very concerned about *MIND's* threat to evict him from the hostel and Jeremy himself is clearly very anxious too. Yesterday, unable to bring himself to read their warning letter he brought it to me to read. Later in the day he called from Paddington station where he had gone, bags packed, to catch a train to Cornwall. He did not go, luckily, but his behaviour shows how agitated he was.

'I am sure he has been aggressive; he acknowledges it himself. But I do not think this matter has been handled very sensibly. Inviting him to attend a rather formal "inquisitorial" meeting is daunting; I am not surprised he did not show up and I will not be surprised if he absents himself today, although I have tried to persuade him to go along calmly. He has a long history of being uncooperative with the professional carers involved in his case - and, goodness knows, there has been a long procession of them, none of them around long enough to build any meaningful or trusting relationship with him. I think it might have been sensible to involve his mother and myself. We have made it very clear that we are involved in his care and have always been so. Indeed I thought it was our right under the CPA to be involved. (Incidentally, in spite of numerous requests on my part, I am still not informed of the dates of CPA review meetings.)

'His present reluctance to engage is compounded by the fact that he has taken against you. I cannot find out for what reason and very likely there is no objective reason, but it does not help the case.

'I am very concerned about what might happen to him were he to be evicted. First of all, it seems to run entirely counter to the whole purpose of the CPA: an all-round package of care. Secondly, (allowing for the fact that the well-being and safety of others is important) it seems somewhat illogical to me to be ready to provide housing for people on Enhanced Care Programmes – itself evidence of their high degree of vulnerability – and then in effect sanction them for suffering from the condition for which they found themselves subject to a care programme in the first place.'

This prompted a phone call from the social worker, who, when I explained my concerns to him, said in that peculiar sanctimonious tone of voice meant obviously to convey empathy but of a neutral non-judgemental variety (God forbid that they should appear to take sides), 'I hear your concern.' I said, 'I know my son can be difficult. *MIND* knows that too but I thought they were in the business of looking after difficult patients... What is more,' I said, 'it is hardly surprising that he should be rather disturbed and on edge himself given that he lives directly above

X with whom he has a history of conflict and who knocked him down the other week as well as setting fire to the place...'

'Oh, oh, I can't say... You can't say... I can't confirm...'

I said, 'I am not asking you to confirm anything. I am telling you what happened, that X set fire to the office. And if you take this into consideration together with the fact that he hit my son so hard he knocked him down, then perhaps it is not really surprising that my son should feel a little unsettled...'

The next day the social worker phoned again to tell me that a Care Plan meeting had been called for Tuesday. 'That's good,' I said, prepared to feel quite well disposed as the man had at least done something. 'What time?' I asked.

'Oh, I can't tell you that.'

'What do you mean you can't tell me? How the hell I am going to be there if you can't tell me the time?'

'Oh, I can't tell you without your son's permission.'

'What?' I said. 'I have been looking after my son for seventeen years, so has his mother. We are his carers. It is our right under the Care Plan. What are you talking about?'

'I can't tell you without your son's consent.'

I put the phone down, apoplectic with rage. I phoned my ex and told her what had happened. She had already received notification of the meeting from the hospital and gave me the time.

It was as much as I could do to keep my hands off the social worker when he arrived. I told the consultant in front of everyone what I felt: that I thought the social worker's behaviour absolutely indefensible, arrogant and stupid. 'How can you hope to build a network of care or any trusting relationship with people who are going to take such a ridiculous attitude? If he had looked at the records he could have seen for himself that I had been present at Care Plan meetings for years.' I said, 'He is just the most recent in a line of social workers so long that I have lost count and forgotten their names. He'll be gone before long for one reason or another and we will still be here, because we have to be.'

The consultant told me firmly that the social worker was only doing his duty and following the rules and that was how it had to be. So I shut up, fuming. If I had not been pretty sure that the consultant shared my views in this matter – not that he ever said so – I would have left the meeting. I said that I trusted that in future both Jeremy's mother and myself would be kept informed of what was going on, as we had been in the past.

As Jeremy seemed so unsettled on his current medication, the decision was taken to increase the dosage. The consultant assured me that even this increased amount was well within the limits of what was permissible. As to the "social" side of Jeremy's life it was found yet again that he did not have any focus to his life, any meaningful activity to occupy his days. This was the key problem "identified" by the social worker. It was decided that he would concentrate on helping Jeremy find such an activity, by joining a writers' group, for example, or signing up for a course. All very laudable and sensible, although why this social worker thought that he was going to succeed where an untold number of predecessors had failed was not clear. They might have got Jeremy involved in something if there had been any continuity in his care, if some one person had stayed in his life long enough to win his confidence.

So Jeremy won a reprieve from the threat of eviction. And the social worker went about encouraging him to sign up for a course, rather successfully as it turned out. Jeremy duly enrolled for a French course – in Toulouse – and stopped accepting his medication. Every time the nurse came round to administer the injection, he either refused or just absented himself. I was not told, presumably in conformity with the social worker's belief in the sacrosanctity of his client's autonomy, although I am the one person who might have been able to persuade him. Jeremy told me himself about some of the occasions on which he had missed the appointment for his injection; he did not tell me that he had had no medication for six weeks when he left for Toulouse.

He organised his enrolment on the course, paid for it, found accommodation and booked a through train ticket. The authorities began to get worried. I was rather proud of him for having managed to set the whole thing up, but I was anxious too. I thought it quite possible he might not get to the train when the day came. It was a ten-day course. I thought it very unlikely he would manage to see the whole thing through. I was anxious more particularly about his accommodation, because he had arranged a room in someone's private house and the man had very kindly said he would come and meet him at the railway station. How could he not notice that there was something pretty strange about my son and then what would happen? I was frightened of what might happen if there were any confrontation.

Yet Jeremy was so determined to go, so determined that he could manage it, I took his part. I took some precautions, however. I knew that one of the best friends of my French psychiatrist cousins, a psychiatric nurse, lived in Toulouse. I contacted her. Then Jeremy's own French cousins lived only two or three hours' drive away. I know Toulouse and I thought, well, even if things do go wrong, it is not far to go.

To my astonishment he managed the trip: Eurostar to Lille and TGV to Toulouse – an all-day journey, without smoking: that perhaps the biggest achievement of all. It was a Sunday. I waited all day with my heart in my mouth. In the evening he phoned to say he had arrived and everything was fine; he was tired and he was going to sleep.

On Monday we had some friends to lunch. We had just sat down to eat when the phone rang. 'That will be Jeremy,' I said. It was. He had been to his school, registered, paid for a fortnight's lessons and spent all morning in the classroom. I was impressed. He wanted me to come out, immediately. 'We could go and see the Médards,' he said; that is his cousins. 'But you have only just started the course,' I said. 'Besides, I can't come just like that.' Then I relented; he was very insistent and sounded a bit desperate. 'I'll see if there are any flights,' I said, 'and I'll call you back.'

I talked to Camilla. 'Go,' she said. 'It's safer. You can always stay there with him.' There was an Easyjet flight the next morning; I booked it. I called Jeremy and told him. He said he would be home from school at two o'clock and would wait for me.

I rented a car at Toulouse airport. Best be prepared, I thought. And I set off to find Jeremy's address, in a quiet sunny street not far from the station. As it was early I walked to the end of the street where I had noticed some shops and stopped at a café to have something to eat and read a paper. I went back to the house about two and rang the bell. There was no reply. I rang repeatedly and still there was no reply. I crossed the street to the far pavement and called his name. Nothing. Stymied. I had no mobile phone in those days; in fact, I think it was that episode that persuaded me against my better judgement to acquire one.

What to do? I found a pay phone but still could not get any reply. I returned to the house and waited. A young man arrived, stood back from the building and yelled up someone's name. A man appeared on a balcony and called down. The first caller crossed the street towards the entrance. Quickly I intercepted him. He said the bell was out of action. 'Come in with me.' He was going to visit a friend lodging in the same flat as Jeremy.

We went up the stairs together and the friend let us in. He showed me Jeremy's room. The door was open and Jeremy was sitting cross-legged and motionless on the bed. At first he scarcely acknowledged me. I saw at once that he was not well. He looked pale, strained and exhausted. He had not been to his classes, he told me. He could not manage it. And it turned out also that there had been some kind of contretemps the previous day. There was a German psychiatrist in the class and it seems – I have never discovered exactly what happened – that Jeremy had had some kind of confrontation with him and was told off by the teacher.

He had had nothing to eat. A fellow lodger – the flat-owner, it seems, let out several rooms to visiting students – had very kindly made him a plate of pasta, but he did not want to eat it.

'Why don't you stay, Dad?' he said.

'Let's go to the Médards first,' I said, 'so you can have a bit of a rest. Besides, I don't really want to have to stay in a hotel for several days.'

'You could stay here.'

'Come on,' I said. 'Let's just get your things together and go to Le Fleix. I told them we were coming. Let's take everything. That way we can decide what to do later.'

At first he seemed willing to leave, to give up any idea of completing the course. It was obvious he could not possibly make it. 'Forget about the cost,' I said. 'It doesn't matter.'

'But I've paid Monsieur X only for one week.'

'It does not matter. He's got a week's money for two days. He is not going to mind. I'll write and explain when we get home.'

'But I want to come back to complete the course.'

'Let's just take everything now and then we can see how you feel when you have had a rest. That way we are free to do what we want.' I did not want to have a confrontation. 'It'll be wonderful to see le Fleix again. You have not been there for years, since Tante Alice died. And Henri is there.'

Henri is the same age as Jeremy. When they were little they used to play together. 'Do you remember that time you crashed on the bikes?'

How old had they been? Seven or eight, maybe. They had got their handlebars entangled speeding down a steep hill and taken an almighty tumble into the ditch. 'It'll be fun to see Henri again. Come on. Let's go. It'll be like having a holiday together.'

I knew he could not possibly stay safely in Toulouse on his own and I did not think my presence there would be much help either. I had to get him home. 'Take the keys with you. We can always post them if necessary.'

We did not say goodbye to anyone. The owner luckily was not at home. Quickly and stealthily we went downstairs and put his things in the car. I had to turn it in the street. Jeremy stood on the pavement and watched me do it. He was standing right beside a metal stanchion, which, in my anxiety, I did not notice. He watched me back into it without saying a word. I got out and looked at the damage. I made no comment. There was a scratch and a slight dent, so small I thought I might get away with it. Already I had decided that I would try, by hook or by crook, to get Jeremy to come home with me. I did not want to do or say anything, which might make that harder to achieve.

It was a relief to be on the road. I phoned our cousins to tell them we were on the way.

They were wonderful and so welcoming. My special friend Jean-François was there with his wife; they were my contemporaries. There were two of their children, Henri and one of his sisters, with Henri's wife, Jeremy's contemporaries, and four or five grandchildren. The house exists for children; there is always a certain hugger-mugger and we were received into it in the most natural way, without any special fuss or attention, as if the house opened its arms to us and closed them round us; we were family and we were taken in. And so little had changed. The interior of the house had been renovated a bit since their old mother had died, but the outhouse remained in the same tumbledown state it had been in the afternoon Jeremy and Henri staggered in bloody and bruised from their collision thirty-five years earlier; the front gate still sagged on its hinge beneath the old rose pergola and the broad green Dordogne, weighted still with snow melt and spring rain, slid powerfully past just across the lane. Eternal, unchanging things: reminders both of happier times and of the transience of human joys and woes.

Jeremy was at ease too. I bought him some beers and he went and sat in the garden to smoke and drink. No one minded or commented if he did not want to sit at table during a meal. They made sure he had what he wanted and left him to do what made him comfortable. But he was not well and that kept me on tenterhooks; I lay awake at night listening for his footsteps above my head, but, mercifully, he seems always to sleep fairly soundly.

I phoned the car hire company to make sure I could hand the car in at Calais. Then we phoned Jeremy's mother who happened to be in Paris that weekend and arranged to meet her. That provided a bait that resolved his lingering doubts about returning to Toulouse.

I had picked him up on a Tuesday. On Thursday morning we set off for Paris. I was so glad that we had stopped at Le Fleix, for that autumn Henri phoned me at home in London to say that his father, Jean-François, had just died of a heart attack. Without Jeremy's little escapade I would not have seen my friend again.

We drove up the autoroute, stopping at the occasional service station for a pee or a coffee and sandwich. Jeremy seemed to enjoy that.

We entered Paris by the Porte d'Italie. I had found a couple of rooms in one of the few remaining old-time hotels, that were basic – lino and shared bathrooms – impeccably clean and cheap. I had to leave the car in an underground park; finding a place on the street is impossible nowadays. We took possession of our rooms and went out to find something to eat. Jeremy was in a dark mood. I do not recall exactly what provoked it, but suddenly he lost his temper and I thought he was going to hit me again. Exhausted by four days of anxiety and tension, I said, probably rather tearfully, as I was at the end of my tether: 'If you do that, I am going to leave you right here. I don't care what happens to you.' He relented and was contrite. We sat and had a beer. What do you talk about in these situations? Schizophrenia makes ordinary inconsequential conversation difficult at the best of times.

We bought some Vietnamese takeaway – eating in a restaurant was out of the question – and went back to the hotel. The night passed without mishap. In the morning I went to call Jeremy, as we had to get to the *Deux Magots*, the famous old literary café in Saint-Germain, to meet his mother for nine o'clock. I said I thought the best thing would be to pack all our things, take the car and then go straight on to Calais. Jeremy announced that he was not going to come with me to London but was going to stay in Paris. I said, 'If we are going to meet your mum we are going to have leave now and catch the métro.' He did not want to go by metro. I said, 'Well, I'm going back to my room to pack my things. You decide.' And with a sinking heart I went back to my room. In a few minutes Jeremy arrived. 'I've been thinking about it, Dad. Let's go home. I'll come with you.' He had his bag in his hand. 'It's better that way, love,' I said. 'I am sure it is.'

We collected the car and drove to the boulevard Saint-Germain. There was an underground car park just opposite the *Deux Magots*. We crossed the street to the café. It was a cold grey morning with not many people about. He did not want to sit inside so we took a table on the *terrasse* facing the boulevard. His mum arrived very soon and we huddled over hot chocolate and *croissants*. I do not know what we talked about, a little chit-chat about our cousins. Jeremy talked French a little with his mum. It was like old times, he said, the three of us... Not a line of conversation I enjoy, but something he does, has always done since the first onset of his illness: this harking back to a time of all being together.

We spent hardly half an hour at the café before setting off for the coast. I did not get away with the scratches to the car; they charged me some astonishing extra amount. We got on the boat, made our way to the station at Dover and caught a train to London. As ill luck would have it, the train became very crowded, filling up with youngsters going into town for Friday night. There was no way of preserving any privacy; we were in an open carriage. A boy aged about sixteen sat down opposite us. His skull was completely shaven. 'Are you a Nazi?' Jeremy said, straight out, by way of conversation. Rather taken aback the boy made some defensive reply. I frowned fiercely at him, trying to discourage him from pursuing the conversation. I do not remember what was said, but voices were raised. I tried to get Jeremy to drop the matter. He said some rather strange, disconnected things. Other passengers standing in the aisle nearby began to take an interest in what was happening. 'What's the matter with you? Are you some kind of nutter?' the boy said. Jeremy told him he was a f*** idiot. 'That's enough,' I said, glowering as disapprovingly as I could at the boy. I tried to persuade Jeremy to swap places with me but he would not. Luckily they both fell silent and the boy got off at a suburban station.

We arrived home. I drove Jeremy back to the hostel. A few days later he was taken to hospital and "sectioned". He had had no medication for six weeks, I discovered.

A couple of years later I referred to that "nightmare journey". 'Don't say that, Dad,' Jeremy replied, somewhat plaintively. 'We had a really nice holiday.'

*

That was May. In July a long anticipated and major improvement took place at the Royal Free: the Grove Centre opened, a new and separate building for the psychiatric wards, in which every patient could have his own room. There were fewer beds, the acoustics were bad, some of the materials used were not as resistant as they needed to be: nonetheless, it was an unalloyed improvement on the old wards. It was a pity that they could not have engaged a sign writer who knew how to spell: a neat plaque above the entrance of Solent Ward announced that this was the departement (*sic*) of psychiatry.

Jeremy was much happier. At least he could retreat to the privacy of his own room with his own washing facilities. He struck up a few friendships, always a bit volatile as I suppose is inevitable with an illness that so disturbs people's perceptions of the world. But, regularly medicated once more, he quickly returned to his normal level of stability.

Chapter Nine
At Last A New Start

After the fiasco of the search for accommodation during the previous hospital admission, I raised the question of where Jeremy was going to live when the time came for discharge in the very first days of this one. He was adamant that he did not want to go back to the *MIND* hostel and they – by "they" I mean their housing management, not the hostel staff – were adamant that they did not want him back. The social worker or the housing adviser – God knows who does what in this complicated bureaucracy – suggested that they should refer Jeremy to an organisation called *New Routes*, whose speciality was "assertive outreach".

The name was encouraging. It suggested that here at last were a bunch of people who understood the difficulties of dealing with patients suffering from schizophrenia, their reluctance or inability to understand or persevere with bureaucratic procedures or indeed engage at all with the "care system": a bunch of people who were prepared to intervene forcefully, if necessary, in order to help patients live successfully "in the community". Of course there were referral procedures to be gone through and then *New Routes* had to assess Jeremy and decide whether they could "take him on": a process, the consultant said, that could take a considerable amount of time. 'How much?' I said. 'Well, months,' he said.

The first signs were not auspicious. I see from a letter I wrote to the social worker on July 17th that *MIND's* housing manager had still – after nearly two months – not completed the procedure for Jeremy's housing application, without which he could not be referred to *New Routes*. She was waiting, she said, for him to come up to the hostel to sign it. A pretty unrealistic expectation in view of the fact that a) he was in hospital and b) she had said she did not want him back in the hostel. I told the social worker that it was precisely this kind of bureaucratic incompetence that had kept my son in hospital so long last time. 'I should be grateful,' I wrote, 'if you would look into this and see that no avoidable delays take place.'

He replied that he was going on a course and would no longer be involved in Jeremy's care. He had arrived on the scene in January or February, heard my concern but kept me at arm's length out of respect for his client's autonomy, unable, without my son's consent, to disclose the time of meetings I had been attending for years, encouraged my son to go on a course which led to my having to go to Toulouse to rescue him and now, in July, after a mere six months of involvement, he was going off on a course and washing his hands of the whole business. Par, one might justly say, for the course!

My son's "section" was lifted in December. In theory he was well enough to return to what is variously called "life in the community" or "mainstream life" where, under the benevolent guidance of the Camden and Islington Mental Health and Social Care Trust, inspired by "therapeutic optimism" and its core principles of "social inclusion" and "recovery", – illness having been abolished and replaced by a "well-being agenda" some time in the course of *anno domini* 2005 – he would once more resume his "journey of recovery" along one of the many possible "flexible pathways" that he could now choose for himself. Unluckily, however, for my son this wonderful adventure in cloudcuckooland could not begin because he was officially homeless, even though I had publicly warned against this danger six months earlier, and therefore could not be discharged from hospital.

On December 27th I wrote to the Chief Executive of the Royal Free:

'My son was admitted to the Royal Free under "section" in May. He suffers from schizophrenia and has done so for seventeen years, during all of which time he has been under the care of the Royal Free. His "section" was lifted a few weeks ago and he has been able to go out on leave. He cannot be discharged, however, because he is homeless and it is the responsibility of the hospital to arrange suitable accommodation for him – something which can take a very long time, as we know to our cost.

'The ward staff let him go out on leave, having no idea where he is going to sleep. Their excuse is that since he is now a voluntary patient they have no power over him. He is not the most co-operative of patients and sometimes keeps in daily touch, sometimes not. When he returns to the hospital he is given a bed sometimes in this room or ward, sometimes in that. Sometimes – tonight, for instance, despite having arranged this morning to sleep on the ward, as he thought – the staff want him to go to Daleham House [about half a mile from the hospital]. Not surprisingly, he finds this uncertainty very disturbing and psychologically unsettling. It is not the kind of treatment that someone with a history of illness like his should be subjected to.

'I am aware of the difficulties faced by the hospital, the pressure on beds and so forth. But my son is a vulnerable patient, he is on an Enhanced Care Plan, his history is well known. It is simply not good enough to shuffle him from pillar to post in this way. Whether or not, strictly speaking, he needs to be in hospital is neither here nor there. He is in hospital and, as long as he is, he is your responsibility. What is the point of getting him well enough to go out into the world again and then treating him in such a way that you could bring on a relapse?

'The Royal Free is a hospital, a place for the care of sick people and no one is more in need of care than the mentally ill. Cutting costs by reducing the number of beds, which is what you have done already in these new wards, or by shuffling patients about as you are doing with my son is... Well, words fail me. It is such a violation of all that any of us ever thought our health service was supposed to be there for.'

I received a reply from the Patient Affairs and Risk Manager, telling me that this matter was now the responsibility of the Camden and Islington Mental Health and Social Care Trust, not the hospital's. I then received a letter from this Trust saying they were "most concerned about the issues" I had raised and had "asked for a thorough, confidential investigation", but would need my son's written consent. I said I was not asking for any personal information about my son; rather I was telling them something about what was happening to my son. Where was the need for anybody's consent?

On February 1st 2006 I received an official 'response to my complaint' informing me that an investigation had been carried out by Mr George Platts (Assistant Locality Director), Ms Danae Dangare, (Lead Nurse), and Mr Dauda Lumeh, (Ward Manager). They found, needless to say, that there was nothing untoward about my son's treatment. They explained how leave from the ward was arranged, how they gave my son medication to take with him and assessed him on his return. There was no reference to my point that they did not know where he was going, that he was in fact crashing out at various girlfriends' places until they chucked him out. Was that a therapeutically suitable arrangement for someone in his condition? They explained that Daleham House was their Rehabilitation Unit – something I have known for twenty years as it is in my street – to which they sent patients well enough but not able to be discharged, completely ignoring my point that this was but one address among many to which he was being sent, randomly and at the last minute, without any preparation, without any consistent programme. And, lastly, they explained: 'the provision of sufficient acute beds in Camden was taken into consideration when the new building was designed. Unfortunately, the problem of bed blockers affects the bed capacity. Mental health services do inevitably end up with various service users who cannot be placed elsewhere for different reasons, after their acute mental health needs have been resolved. In most cases the problem is actually not the responsibility of the Mental Health Services as other agencies are usually organising their housing needs.'

Of course! It is always someone else's responsibility. And might not the "inevitability" of "ending up with various service users" have been taken into consideration too, when designing the new building, which in any case was designed to house fewer patients than the old Royal Free wards? Why was it designed for fewer patients, especially in view of the fact, as we are continually reminded, that Camden has one of the most difficult problems with mental illness in the country? Was it because the powers-that-be foresaw a decrease in the numbers of patients with "mental health needs" or because they had an eye on their account books? And what, one might ask, was their "evidence base," as the jargon now goes? And why are Mental Health Services capitalised in one sentence and not in another? Patients called patients in one sentence and service users in another? And we thought there was supposed to be a joined-up system, a "seamless network of care"!

I wrote again to the Trust's Chief Executive on February 14th. Jeremy was still being shuffled from pillar to post.

'Last night,' I wrote, 'my son phoned me at about 9pm to tell me that there was no bed for him on Solent Ward (his regular ward at the new Grove Centre) and could he come here. Well, he had been staying with me and before that, on and off, with a friend who then told him she wanted him to leave. In the event he slept here. He was quite happy to sleep on Solent Ward but they told him he would have to go to St Pancras [another hospital a mile away] and, quite understandably, he did not want to.

'This is not a satisfactory state of affairs and not good for his health. I want to know exactly whose responsibility it is to find him a place to live and when they are going to do it. The situation is absurd... He spent a whole year at the Royal Free in 2002 because no one would find him a place to live.'

In fact the situation was more than absurd. For while all this was going on my son's old room in the *MIND* hostel remained empty – and was being paid for – because it could not be re-let until my son had been re-housed!

I wrote also to the ward manager, the person most immediately responsible for my son's sleeping arrangements. I received no reply. I wrote also to my son's consultant, whom I knew to be unhappy at what was going on.

This is what he wrote:

'I was sorry to hear of your on-going concerns about Jeremy's current situation, with which I must say I have a lot of sympathy. I was very surprised to learn that you have already received a reply to your complaint to our Trust's Chief Executive, because I was not even told about it by the managers involved, let alone being asked to comment on the issues you raised. This will confirm for you that I actually have very little influence over Jeremy's current situation regarding his protracted stay in the Grove Centre or his obtaining a new flat in the local area.

'...it was in June 2005 that I first suggested to our Multi-Disciplinary Team that Jeremy should be referred to the *New Routes* Team, and that at the same time measures should be taken to end his tenancy with *Mind in Camden* and to obtain a flat for him in the North Camden area. As I have recently discovered, in actual fact, all of this was postponed, on the assumption that these measures would be undertaken by the *New Routes* Team when they eventually started working with Jeremy.

'As you know, *New Routes* did not complete their assessment of Jeremy until recently, at which point he refused to have anything more to do with them... [*New Routes*, remember, specialise in "*assertive* outreach" (my emphasis)]

'Currently Jeremy's housing situation is being addressed by the Hospital Link Worker attached to the Housing Department... She continues to liaise with the manager of *New Routes*... and we are planning to convene a CPA meeting... in the near future... to share views and ideas about how to improve Jeremy's situation. I should be happy if you could attend. You would also have the opportunity to meet Jeremy's new CPA care-coordinator... (yes – yet another change of personnel which has nothing to do with me!).

'Finally, to end on yet another negative note. Pressure on beds at the Grove Centre and in the other psychiatric in-patient units in Camden is ever-increasing. Although I have previously asked that Jeremy should NOT be obliged to move to other wards or units in order to make way for newly-admitted patients... I doubt that my request will be heeded for much longer. There is a strong possibility that Jeremy will be asked to re-locate temporarily to another ward or even to a "bed & breakfast" hotel paid for by the Grove Centre.'

In the meantime the Mental Health Trust acquired a new chief executive. She it was who replied to my letter of February 14th: 'I was most concerned about the issues you have raised and I have asked for a thorough, confidential investigation...' – identical words to the reply to my letter of December 27th. A month later, on March 20th, she wrote again to say that the investigation was "taking slightly longer than anticipated". I do not think I was ever told what the investigation had revealed, and I do not suppose I missed much. However, on that same day, Camden's Housing Needs Group Quality and Review Officer, Damien Dwyer, wrote to Glenda Jackson, who had once more intervened on our behalf. He explained to Glenda Jackson that 'a number of housing options *appear* [my emphasis] to have been considered...' and 'a number of staff and organisations have been involved in the discussions...' In listing them, he called their own organisation *New Routes* New Roots and got the name of Jeremy's consultant wrong. Then he attributed the responsibility for nothing having been achieved to Jeremy's 'not being agreeable to some of the proposals.' (How assertive does an Assertive Outreach Team have to be to win the accolade "Assertive"?)

He went on to explain that Jeremy, now in a compliant phase, had 'an application to the Council's Allocations scheme and is able to bid for studio accommodation. He has 205 points with which to bid'.

'Since Jeremy has been able to bid, eighteen studio properties have been let under the choice-based allocations scheme. Of these, three were let for less than 205, with a further three let for less than 230 points.

'...there is not a great deal of information yet available about the amount of points required to successfully bid for certain categories of property. Yet it appears clear from the foregoing information that Jeremy has less than the average number of points required to bid successfully for a studio property, and that he will therefore need to bid frequently and for a wide variety of properties in order to place a successful bid in the near future. It seems reasonably clear, in addition, however, that Jeremy has grounds for hope that he will be able to obtain accommodation in the near future, if he is willing to consider a wide range of properties...'

We are talking about a person who has been suffering for nearly twenty years from an extremely disabling condition. Why does he have only 205 points, when need is supposed to be the criterion according to which points are allocated? What use are

205 points if they are not really sufficient to allow you to compete in this auction, this bidding lottery? As for the bidding process and expecting someone with a history of schizophrenia to cope with it...

It goes something like this: you have to get a copy of the *Camden New Journal* every week, find the accommodation vacant pages, find the properties that fall within your points range, ring a telephone number, key in a PIN number and a reference for the property you wish to compete for. You do not speak to any human person. You have not seen the property. You then wait to hear whether your bid has been successful enough to win you the right to take an actual look at what you have bid for...

'It seems reasonably clear... that Jeremy has grounds for hope that he will be able to obtain accommodation in the near future, if he is willing to consider a wide range of properties,' wrote the Quality Review Officer. "seems", "reasonably clear", "grounds for hope", "near future", "if", "willing to consider", "wide range of properties": is that encouraging or isn't it? What sort of odds would a bookmaker give you if you represented your chances to him in that sort of language?

And let us not even imagine what kind of property might be available in that 'wide range,' so wide that with a below-average 205 points you might have a vague chance of picking up the scraps that nobody else wanted. A nice secluded spot on a nice quiet housing estate, with peaceful, polite and understanding neighbours: somewhere private where you will not be exposed to a lot of noisy teenagers and other phenomena that you might find threatening? It does not seem very likely. In fact, I find it rather shocking that a Council employee could entertain such propositions, apparently, without a flicker of embarrassment, without a shadow of awareness of the bitter irony in what he was describing.

But there was a silver lining: Peter Beadle, the new care-coordinator and community psychiatric nurse whom the consultant had mentioned in his letter turned out to be one of the best we have ever had. First of all, he got in touch with me immediately to tell me he was taking over. But, most important, he managed to build a relationship with Jeremy such that Jeremy would phone him, meet with him, talk with him quite willingly. It was not to last of course; he was to leave, but he was there for a year and a half and helped us through a difficult transition.

*

There was no progress in the search for somewhere for Jeremy to live. He did make one or two bids, but nothing came of them. It was clear that he was not going to be able to keep up the sort of relentless endeavour necessary to produce any result and that *New Routes* were far too spineless to be any help. It was equally clear that the chances of finding somewhere nice were very remote. I was going to have to do it again.

I sold the old flat. The freeholder, who occupied the two lower floors, had asked me several times if I would sell him the top floor. He was only too keen to buy, so we got a good price. The government of course took 40% of the difference between the price I had bought at fifteen years ago and the price I sold at. House prices had risen enormously in the meantime, so I had proportionally less money to spend on a new flat. I began to house-hunt, with the usual disappointments; you see dozens of shoddy over-priced conversions and places that are completely unsuitable. I found one on a local housing estate, ex-Council, low-rise, spacious, with a balcony and view of grass and trees. We checked it out at night to make sure it was safe and quiet. My offer was accepted; everything seemed to be going ahead, when the owner cried off. I had to start again.

Then a friend put me in touch with a local estate agent. I explained that we needed somewhere above all safe and quiet; I did not tell him exactly what the circumstances were, because you never know how people will react. He was extremely kind and helpful and found me somewhere nearby. We made an offer. The owner lived somewhere in the Gulf states, could not be contacted easily. Eventually we heard that our offer was accepted. Then nothing happened for a while. It looked as if this one too was going to change his mind. The estate agent persuaded him this was an opportunity he should not let slip and finally the place was ours. It was October.

Jeremy had known for a few months that I was trying to buy him a flat. I had had to tell him when I thought I was buying the ex-Council flat; I wanted him to have a look at it. So he had abandoned any attempt to find a place through the Council's "allocations scheme", although his points allocation had finally been raised to 305. I told the consultant too at a ward round, but warned him that I would have to carry out some alterations before Jeremy could move in. So plans were made to prepare for him to leave hospital in January 2007. For the first few months he would not be formally discharged but considered to be on extended leave. *New Routes* would support him. There was one support worker he liked and who seemed to have convinced him that trying cognitive behavioural therapy might be helpful. As usual, as soon as Jeremy had decided that he would co-operate with this man he left.

We started work on the flat. The more time I spent in it, the more I felt it was a good place, the right place for Jeremy. It was much smaller than his previous flat: just one large room, with a separate small kitchen and bathroom. But it was purpose-built with solid floors, so less chance of noise from neighbours. There was no one above. It faced south, overlooking an internal garden quadrangle. There were lovingly maintained gardens all around. There were a number of mildly eccentric, even slightly dotty, people among the residents, so looking not entirely conventional would not draw particular attention. It was in a safe, respectable neighbourhood, close to shops, close to me as well as to his mother.

By New Year 2007 everything was ready. I had fetched Jeremy's books and personal things back from my brother's, where they had been in store for five years. Jeremy moved in, I think, on January 4th 2007. I was anxious, worried about his reaction to the neighbours as usual, but fairly confident that he was well enough to stand a good chance of living here successfully.

And so it has turned out. He has settled quite comfortably and easily into a new life in his flat. There are numerous shops and cafés nearby, so getting supplies is easy. One of the cafés has become a kind of home from home. He still does not risk sitting inside very often, but he has made friends there and he announced with some pride the other day that the six or seven people I had seen sitting around him outside a local pub were all friends. 'I have got a circle of friends now, Dad.'

There is indeed a real sense in which he has begun to build something more substantial for himself than he has ever managed before. His moods remain changeable and there are still periods when he takes against me and will not speak to me, but they do not last very long and he is much better than ever before at talking about and explaining both what is going on and things that have happened in the past.

*

The difficulties we have encountered this time have been of a practical and bureaucratic nature, nothing to do with Jeremy's state of health.

The first was Housing Benefit. In Jeremy's old flat the London Borough of Camden had paid his rent to me in the form of Housing Benefit even though I was the father. I had taken the precaution of checking with them that they were still prepared to do this. In the old flat they had paid £209 a week, out of a commercial rate of £220, i.e. 95%; that was in 2001. I assumed that they would pay at least the same amount or the same proportion now. Estate agents told me the going market rent for the new flat would be £220 a week, the same, as it happens, as for the former flat six years ago.

We duly applied for Housing Benefit. To my surprise Jeremy's entitlement was assessed at only £165 per week. These decisions are made on the basis of a formula involving what they call claim-related rent and average rents for similar types of accommodation in the same neighbourhood. I wrote to say that I thought this assessment was most unfair, especially in view of the fact that they had been prepared to pay 95% of the commercial rent six years previously and that both the advice of estate agents in the area and internet property searches showed that a decent studio flat for under £200 per week was impossible to find. Anything cheaper would be very small, often with a kitchen that was part of the living-sleeping area and just a shower for a bathroom. 'My son is not an ordinary tenant,' I said, 'he has been disabled by schizophrenia since finishing university nearly twenty years ago. He has never been able to have a job. He spends most of his life in his flat... The room he sleeps and spends most of his day in is around 4m by 5m. Is he not entitled to a space this size to spend his life in?' I said I did not expect them to pay the full market rent but that I thought something in the region of £185 per week would be fairer.

A week later, on March 8th, they wrote to my son telling him that his father had queried his Housing Benefit assessment, but that they had not replied directly to me because they did not have his written permission to do so. They proposed two options to him. One was to seek a re-determination of the rent officer's decision, but they forgot to fill in the amounts which he was being invited to disagree with: "£[Click here and type amount]", their letter said. The other was to apply for a Discretionary Housing Payment (with an application form to fill in, of course). 'If I do not receive your written reply in this office **within One Month of the date of this letter** [their emphasis] I will presume that you no longer wish to dispute the decision on your claim.' The date was March 8th.

I received no reply to the letters I had written on March 1st and March 2nd, not even to tell me that they could not deal directly with me without my son's authorisation. My son did not tell me about the March 8th letter with the one-month deadline until March 26th; he had not even opened it himself.

I wrote again. I reiterated my arguments and pointed out that the cost of keeping someone in hospital for three years because the "system" failed to find him somewhere to live and then paying for his room in a hostel to remain empty for eighteen months, thus at the same time also depriving someone else of a place to live when there was already a shortage of such accommodation, must have been ludicrously expensive. And now they were quibbling about paying what they had been happy to pay several years earlier when all the responsibility of maintenance and so on would be mine.

They replied that they had "noted the contents" of my letter; 'however, this does not change the situation, as we still need a reply to the letter sent to your son on 8 March'. This time they enclosed a copy of that letter for me, but this time they had filled in the figures missing from the original they had sent to my son.

And so, tediously, it went on. I got my son to write a note authorising me to act on his behalf. I appealed to Glenda Jackson for help. And, miraculously, on May 4th I received a letter from Camden Finance Department telling me that we had been awarded a Discretionary Housing Payment, that the Rent Officer had been asked to look again at his assessment and that, whatever the outcome of that re-determination turned out to be, we would receive an overall amount of £220 per week to cover Jeremy's rent. Five months to sort that one out. Discretionary payments are of course only discretionary, which means that we have to go through the performance of re-applying year by year, living always with the possibility that the answer might be no.

I also wrote to the Minister of State for Health, Rosie Winterton, pointing out that this sort of bureaucratic difficulty over something as important to people's health as housing hardly fitted the policy of providing a "seamless network of care" for the mentally ill. The reply, most conveniently: this is the responsibility of the Department of Work and Pensions, not us.

There were similar problems with Disability Living Allowance and Income Support. The procedures are unbelievably bureaucratic and further complicated by the fact that so much of the correspondence is generated automatically by computers, so that, for example, every communication relating to Income Support starts by telling you that due to "a change in circumstances..." when in fact nothing has changed at all. At first this is worrying, especially when the payments vary, particularly, as in Jeremy's case, after being in hospital for so long that everything has to be worked out afresh; you try to understand what is going and, actually, it is not possible.

It is a frustrating and time-consuming business trying to ensure that someone is receiving the right amount of benefit. In addition to the voluminous correspondence I had to make numerous phone calls. Because of Jeremy's new address we now dealt with Blackpool for the DLA and Glasgow for Income Support. Formerly we had dealt with a Belfast office, where I encountered endless bloody-mindedness. For the people I dealt with in Blackpool and Glasgow I have nothing but praise; they are unfailingly cheerful, courteous and accommodating. Even so it took from January to May to get Jeremy's DLA restarted; it had been suspended while he was in hospital. His CPN undertook to do it at first, but it requires real persistence and a willingness to spend a lot of time waiting for phone calls to go through if you are to make any progress. You need to be confident and forceful too, for the system's left hand often has little idea what it's right hand has been up to. Eventually someone takes pity on you and says, 'Look, I've found the file. We have a terrible backlog, that's the problem. I'll put it on the top of the pile and it will be dealt with on Monday or Tuesday...' And it is.

Yet almost at once further problems arise. The government is, sensibly enough, trying to reduce fraudulent claims for disability allowances, so Jeremy is summoned to attend for a medical examination in some other part of London. How is he going to get there? Is he going to keep the appointment? What will happen if he does not? He has just spent the best part of three years in hospital. Is that not by itself sufficient evidence of his disability? I write to object, the care co-ordinator also; we produce statements signed by doctors and the matter is cleared up.

Then it is necessary to re-apply for Disability Living Allowance. The form comprises thirty-nine pages of questions. Do you need someone with you to guide or supervise you when walking outdoors in unfamiliar places? Tick the appropriate box: 1) to avoid danger; 2) I may get lost or wander off; 3) I have anxiety or panic attacks; 4) to make sure I am safe.

Which category does feeling your knees crunch and having to return home come under? Or being too scared to go and fetch a prescription? And how many days a week do you need this help? Can you say? What if it is only occasionally?

Do you need help from another person or do you have difficulty washing, bathing, showering or looking after your appearance? And how many days a week? What are you to say? I am a dirty scruff and seldom shave or change my clothes?

Would you have difficulty preparing and cooking a main meal for yourself? Caution: this does not mean reheating ready-made meals or convenience foods. Tick the box: 1) I have difficulty planning a meal; 2) I lack the motivation to cook...

I'll say! And how many days a week? And does ticking the box mean that you will get any help with preparing a meal? Assuming that you are able to say this kind of thing about yourself time and again over thirty-nine pages.

I had, of course, to get yet more consent forms signed. However, I found the attitude of these DWP employees much more sensible and responsible than in local government and the Mental Health Trust: they would at least exercise some discretion and agree to speak to you and provide non-personal information.

The biggest headache was Income Support. Jeremy's new care-coordinator, Peter, had warned me that he thought the DWP might try to make Jeremy repay the Income Support he had continued to receive during the first months of his last hospital admission.

You are supposed to inform the authorities when you are admitted to hospital and Jeremy had not done so. My argument was, that it was extremely unrealistic to expect someone with schizophrenia, least of all when in the throes of a relapse, to deal with such a bureaucratic issue as this. If it was anybody's responsibility, it should have been the social worker's or the hostel's or even the ward's, all of whom must have been or should have been aware of the procedures to be followed when someone is admitted to hospital "not in his right mind".

I also pointed out that psychiatric admissions are not like ordinary admissions. For one thing they tend to be much longer, but also for much of the time a patient, apart from sleeping on the ward, can go about the business of his life pretty much as usual; Jeremy was out and about all day, buying his usual supplies of tobacco, feeding himself on the usual takeaway food, incurring, in other words, his usual expenses.

A year had gone by and I was beginning to think that Peter's representations that in the circumstances it was not fair to insist on this repayment might have had their effect. But no: while I was out of the country in early 2008 Jeremy told me on the phone that the DWP had reduced his weekly Income Support, claiming that he had been overpaid to the tune of more than £4,600. They told him they were going to pay themselves back at the rate of £9 a week over the next ten years! I advised Jeremy to get his new care co-ordinator – yes, another new one by this time – to act on his behalf.

When I returned home I found that the care co-ordinator had merely listened to the DWP's arguments and repeated them to Jeremy: he had not acted in any way as an advocate for Jeremy. I wrote to the Debt Centre Manager, appealing against this decision, once more copying the correspondence to Glenda Jackson. At the end of April they wrote to say that they were reversing their decision: they had decided there was no longer a case for claiming overpayment on the grounds of failure to disclose information. Needless to say, the system continued to generate bumph as though there had been no change of decision. A few more phone calls were necessary before this problem too could be confined to the archive.

But, again, if I had not intervened and the claim for overpayment of Income Support had been left to the "professionals", my son would have suffered a weekly deduction from his "income" for ten years. Can that be right?

And there were problems with the electricity supply to the flat, confusion over who was supposed to be the supplier, caused entirely by incompetence at EDF and British Gas. Bailiffs were sent round, money was deducted from my account that had to be reimbursed, mail sent to the wrong address... the by now familiar bureaucratic glitches entailed by the corner-cutting mentality of the privatised utility companies.

Obviously this cannot be blamed on the Department of Health. Nonetheless, one wants to ask, how is a person disabled by schizophrenia to cope with the bureaucratic confusion and the complicated procedures involved in just making sure that the fundamental needs of his life are met? A "care package" for serious mental illness that does not include a reliable provision for ensuring that these routine, everyday needs are properly met is not worth the name.

*

What is supposed to happen? Does anyone know? I do not, even after twenty years of involvement.

Locally, it would appear, our fate lies in the hands of our Trust: the Camden and Islington Mental Health and Social Care

Trust, newly reborn as the Camden and Islington NHS Foundation Trust. It announces the birth of a brave new world, a shiny new phoenix that will rise from the pyre of the old with a whole new seductive language at its disposal – a New Speak, as one might say, taking a leaf from "a new build" and "a big ask" – and one that miraculously comes with a price tag eight million pounds cheaper than its predecessor.

The formal discharge from Jeremy's May 2005 admission to hospital took place in June 2007. Sadly we had to say goodbye to the consultant who had played such a large part in getting him well again, his job axed in the Trust's £8 million budget cut, but at least Jeremy was being handed over to another community psychiatrist whom we all knew well and liked. *New Routes*, of whose "assertive" role the Trust makes so much in its attempts to gloss over the difficulties likely to arise from the closure of day hospitals and day centres, sent a representative to the meeting – yet another one, whom none of us had seen before (how do they hope to build trusting relationships with difficult patients when there is no continuity of staff?). Why had he come? He introduced himself and told us that he had been sent along to the meeting to announce that *New Routes* was also discharging Jeremy.

That was not very diplomatic, I suggested: the organisation which is supposed to provide close support turning up at a discharge meeting, in itself a potentially difficult and sensitive moment in a patient's life, and announcing that it is abandoning the person it was supposed to be helping. 'That augurs well,' I said, 'for the Trust's brave new world of modernised, streamlined care.'

So Jeremy moved into his flat without the support of the advertised specialists in providing help to difficult patients with a tendency either not to co-operate with or even drop completely off the radar of the mental health services. Shortly afterwards we lost the care-co-ordinator as well; he moved to another authority, because he was fed up with the changes being introduced as part of the Trust's cost-cutting exercises.

There was no organised hand-over, no introductions. When he left on a Friday, we had no idea who the replacement taking over on the Monday was going to be. And anyway the replacement did not bother to introduce himself, until after I had complained to the Trust that it was not following its own procedures.

Jeremy quickly decided he did not like him and told him so. He was soon replaced by another co-ordinator, who, I am glad to say, has managed to establish good relations with Jeremy. However, she has just informed us that because Jeremy has registered with a new GP practice nearer to where he now lives he comes under the jurisdiction, as it were, of a different Community Mental Health Team. Although both teams, the old and the new, work in the same building, he will have to have another new care co-ordinator as well as a new consultant. That makes four care co-ordinators and three consultants in under two years. I have written to the Trust suggesting that perhaps a good therapeutic relationship is more important than whether a patient receives his fortnightly injection on the ground floor or the first floor. I have received no reply.

Chapter Ten
An Unholy Alliance

An unholy alliance has formed these last few years between providers of care like the Camden and Islington NHS Foundation Trust and the lobbying organisations like *Rethink*, the mental health charity formerly known as the National Schizophrenia Fellowship, which was set up by parents of people suffering from schizophrenia to represent and campaign on behalf of their suffering children. The wolf and the wolfhound have lain down together, as it were. They speak the same language and, unfortunately, the party that suffers are the people with schizophrenia. It is instructive to look at how this has come about.

Existing provisions for looking after the mentally ill are not sufficient; our own experience makes that abundantly clear. Yet our Care Trust plans to cut £8 million from its budget. Three of the five Day Hospitals are to go and the remaining two will become "Recovery Centres"; Day Centres will go; outpatient services are being reduced and community psychiatry posts lost; already there are fewer in-patient beds. When, on June 17th 2007, I wrote to the Chief Executive expressing my alarm at hearing of these cuts she replied that, on the contrary, the Trust's reforms would bring significant benefits. 'Underpinning these developments,' she wrote, 'is a fresh approach to service delivery encapsulated in *the principles of recovery and social inclusion...*' (my emphasis). In a further letter (Aug 8th 2007) she wrote: 'The recovery and social inclusion agenda are very much part of the Care Trust's central plan for it's (*sic*) mental health services... In order to deliver this agenda the Care Trust have had to take some very difficult decisions regarding the present configuration of it's (*sic*) community and day care provision...' (Code for closing various facilities.)

'Finally,' she conceded, 'I can appreciate that in some quarters there is a degree of frustration concerning social inclusion and the recovery model, however the Care Trust are committed to the ethos and ideals that it encompasses and will continue to promote the model as the core approach to working with vulnerable individuals experiencing the effects of mental ill health...'

Reading language like this, I do not think the problem is so much frustration as total incomprehension. How do you deliver an agenda? Can models be approaches? Can models encompass ideals, let alone an ethos? And what is one to make of the shift from talking about service users and clients – offensive but by now familiar terms – to talking about "working with vulnerable individuals experiencing the effects of mental ill health"? She used to talk about mental illness and the mentally ill. Now, quite suddenly, these terms have been dropped; she writes, not of my son's' illness, but of his "recovery journey". These shifts of language are not fortuitous: something is afoot.

When I asked her what was new about "recovery" – 'Isn't recovery, making people better, the whole point of medicine anyway?' – she referred me to the website of the Social Care Institute for Excellence (a title which, one might think, itself begs a few questions): www.scie.org.uk/publications/positionpapers. Here I found a paper entitled "A Common Purpose: Recovery in future mental health services" (sponsored by the Royal College of Psychiatrists, the Care Services Improvement Partnership and the Social Care Institute for Excellence). Its cover photo is of prayer lamps from a temple in Tamil Nadu, India, an illustration, we are told, of *aarti*, "the auspicious lighting of lamps", chosen 'because it carries a wealth of connections and associations with people of all cultures who have created and sustained light, often in dark places, as a harbinger of hope and a symbol of reaching beyond our suffering and limitations'.

Why "the auspicious lighting of lamps" should carry any connections or associations for Welsh, Scottish, Irish, English or indeed any people not Hindus is not made clear.

And for those of us who might be feeling 'a degree of frustration concerning social inclusion and the recovery agenda', the website includes the following:

'There is not yet a succinct or universally accepted definition of recovery. In ordinary speech, recovery is often equated with cure, a return to how things were before the illness or injury occurred, a process of getting back to normal, but by this definition few, if any, who experience severe mental illness recover (Whitwell 2005). However, for severe mental health problems, and in reality all long-term conditions, outcomes are more complex and are described both by resolution of symptoms, impacts on life domains affected by illness, and growth and development of other valued life experiences. Some professional definitions of recovery distinguish between "complete clinical recovery", with total absence of symptoms, and "social recovery", which means the ability to live a more or less independent life even if symptoms remain. The current concept of recovery includes both of these but has moved from professional definitions towards self-definition, such that the concept and experience of personal recovery is not limited by the presence or absence of symptoms, and disabilities, nor the ongoing use of services. The concept of personal recovery pivots around considerations of how to live and how to live well in the context of long-term mental health conditions. How to develop a strong and satisfactory personal identity that is not defined by illness is a key issue, for example: "just because you have a diagnosis of schizophrenia doesn't mean that you have to be a schizophrenic". This way of thinking about recovery engages with the seemingly paradoxical assertion that you can be well even if you have a long-term illness, or as the Stanford University self-management course put it, "Living a healthy life with chronic conditions" (Cooper and Clarke, 2005). Thus recovery has been defined as, "a deeply personal, unique process of changing one's attitudes, values, feelings, goals, skills and roles. It is a way of living a satisfying, hopeful, and contributing life even with limitations caused by the illness. Recovery involves the development of new meaning and purpose in one's life as one grows beyond the catastrophic effects of mental illness (Anthony, 1993)."

In short, put crudely, you do not need to be well to be called well. And if that looks suspiciously like what we used to think of as contradictory, well, just think about it differently: the paradox is illusory. Come back, Maharishi. Light a few candles. Chant a few chants. Maybe there is even a role for the astrologer again. 'Concepts of recovery,' we are told, 'emphasise the value and uniqueness of each person and regard their different viewpoints and cultural perspectives as a resource'.

One can see why such an approach might be attractive to a cash-strapped authority: patients do not need to recover in order to have recovered. Better still, if they do not think they are ill in the first place...! Positive outcomes by the barrelful for your audit.

*

Rather more distressing has been the transformation of the National Schizophrenia Fellowship. Founded in 1971 by the parents of children with schizophrenia in order to campaign for better treatment, it had its name changed to *Rethink* in 2001 on the grounds that the presence of the word schizophrenia in its title attracted stigma and deterred both donors and people who might benefit from its help. A rather surprising point of view, one might think, for an organisation founded by and for people with such an intimate connection with schizophrenia.

In fact it did more than change its name; it was "re-branded". From being an accessible, loose association of people brought together on equal terms by the common experience of schizophrenia, it reinvented itself as a service-provider manned by professional bureaucrats with careers to think about and with little personal knowledge of schizophrenia. In effect, the bureaucrats, taking advantage of a weak chairman, carried out a putsch. It was dressed up as the choice of the majority of members, but as the president of the organisation, commenting on the decision of the Board of Trustees, wrote to me at the time: 'The total number who voted, about 1050 [out of a membership of 7,500], represented 14% of the membership, those in favour of change amounting to 9% of the membership. There was no consensus on the proposed names *Reason* and *Rethink*. 32% of respondents preferred *Reason* and 38% wanted *Rethink*. In both cases a majority of members did not like the proposed names. In the event, the Board chose *Rethink*, a name preferred by 5% of the total membership.' A sympathetic member of staff, who asked to remain anonymous, wrote to say that the balance of power within the organisation had shifted: the professionals had gained the upper hand.

*

Under their influence *Rethink* has become an umbrella organisation for mental illness as a whole, like *MIND*. It makes a periodic show of maintaining a foot in the land of schizophrenia, because it knows that the majority of its members still come from there, but it reveals its real interest in the frequent bandying about of that idiotic statistic of one in four people in this country suffering from "some kind of mental health problem in the course of a year".

The number of people suffering from schizophrenia is between 0.5 and one per cent of the population, depending on the diagnostic system used. If the one-in-four statistic is to mean anything at all it must include routine depression, grief at bereavement, despondency on winter Sundays and disappointment at being passed over for promotion. These are not pathological conditions. Yet time and again in its literature and its proclamations *Rethink* assimilates "some kind of mental health problem" and "severe mental illness". A leaflet designed to recruit new members states: 'A staggering 1 in 4 people in the UK will experience some kind of mental health problem in the course of a year. It's a huge number of people, but, because severe mental illness remains "largely hidden" and shrouded in prejudice, ignorance and fear, most people are unaware of how much distress is being caused to so many...' Thus, "severe mental illness" and "some kind of mental health problem" become co-terminous, co-extensive categories. Thus, feeling so distressed by the unruly behaviour of your fourth-year English class that you cannot face going into school on Monday morning and drowning yourself in the Thames because you can no longer stand the torment of believing that you are being pursued by Nigerian gangsters bent on injecting poison into your blood stream become equivalent.

Lots of people recover from anxieties like those of the English teacher or from bouts of depression induced by desertion or bereavement and are restored, without lasting ill effect, to their normal lives. Thus, *Rethink* can boast how Sophie X, with the help of *Rethink*, overcame depression and stress at work and set up her own business and the Chief Executive can claim confidently that "the three biggest mental health problems in this country today" are "prejudice, ignorance and fear".

There are a number of things one could say about all of this. First, there undoubtedly is prejudice about mental illness, about any kind of "breakdown". And is it not only natural that people should be wary of those who at times do or say odd, strange things, who are a bit "bonkers"? We all recognise it when we hear it or see it. Perhaps sometimes a brief, transient period of oddness is quite without significance, is not in any way evidence of a chronic condition or impairment of the mind, the reason, the ability to function normally, in which case it obviously is unfair to discriminate against people on these grounds. However, there are breakdowns, albeit perhaps not amounting to a "condition", which are serious enough to justify doubts about the subject's ability to perform at full capacity. My father, for instance, had a breakdown. I do not think there was ever any diagnosis of a condition, but it was bad enough for him not to know his own name or recognise his wife, until a couple of bouts of ECT seemed to restore him to normality. He did eventually find a job again, in quite a senior and responsible position, though probably not as senior as he might have achieved had he never had a breakdown. I do not know to what extent, if at all, he concealed the seriousness of what had happened. But surely a prospective employer, contemplating giving a senior position to someone with a history like this, would be acting irresponsibly if he did not take the history into consideration. Is that prejudice? And is the problem the prejudice or the breakdown?

It is also true that people suffering from some serious and chronic conditions, like manic depression, can nonetheless continue to function pretty effectively when properly medicated. For several years I wrote books with a co-author who suffered from manic depression. When she was well, she was as lively, sharp and witty as anyone could wish. I had an uncle who was a high-powered civil servant and took medication for manic depression all his life.

Schizophrenia is a different category of illness. Very few people recover from schizophrenia in the sense that they are able to hold any jobs at all, let alone ones that reflect their true ability; very few are able to maintain ordinary emotional relationships like marriage or to bring up a family. They very often look strange, act strangely, speak strangely, respond strangely, not to say unpredictably, to others. These may not be reasons for not showing compassion and understanding, but it is very far from the truth that they are prevented from recovering, from returning to normal life by stigma and discrimination, by the fear, prejudice and ignorance of others. The problem with schizophrenia is quite clearly schizophrenia, the illness; to pretend otherwise is a foolish, even dangerous, distraction.

But if you conflate the categories of "some kind of mental health problem", "severe mental illness" and "schizophrenia" in this woolly-minded manner it is easy to see how, with some help from bad grammar and a cavalier attitude to the meaning of words, you can end up deceiving yourself into believing that people are not really ill, but merely on a "journey of recovery" with only a few easily surmountable obstacles barring the way to "well-being", as it is now to be called.

The "ethos of Recovery" or the "ethos of optimistic realism", as Paul Farmer, now CEO of *MIND*, used to call it in the days when he was *Rethink*'s Director of Public Affairs, has a nice ring to it: you can imagine someone trying it out for the first time in front of the mirror. It suggests philosophical profundity, intellectual respectability, which no doubt is one of the principal reasons for its being adopted as the rallying cry of professional caring. The fact that ethos does not really have the meaning intended is a minor detail. Words are there to serve our purpose. 'To change social attitudes the terminology has to change.' Thus, a contributor to *Rethink*'s magazine *Your Voice* (winter 2003). He also wrote: 'So far as those diagnosed as "schizophrenic" are concerned, the label is iatrogenic (*sic*) in effect – that is to say that the term itself contributes to the condition it purports to describe.' Does he mean that the boy who was tormented to death by the fear of Nigerian poisoners need not have died? That we contributed to his death by calling him schizophrenic? *Rethink*'s chairman at the time of the name change said she was surprised that I, a writer, did not seem to understand that 'words were vessels to be filled with meaning'.

It would be no bad thing if, along with their equality and diversity training, new staff were made to have a look at the appendix on the Principles of Newspeak in George Orwell's *1984*. 'The purpose of Newspeak was not only to provide a medium of expression for the world-view and mental habits proper to the devotees of Ingsoc, but to make all other modes of thought impossible.' The goal was to make a 'heretical thought – that is, a thought diverging from the principles of Ingsoc – ... literally unthinkable, at least so far as thought is dependent on words'. Words are deliberately constructed for a political purpose, 'intended to impose a desirable mental attitude upon the person using them.' *Rethink*, in what purports to be an interview with Diane Abbott MP (*Your Voice*, autumn 2007), asks, without a trace of misgiving, never mind irony, what the government can do to ensure that mental health services are "culturally sound".

Of Recovery, *Rethink* has this to say: 'There are probably as many definitions of recovery as there are people affected by mental illness but as the ethos has been strongly driven by the user/survivor movement perhaps it is to that body we should look... '

On one level one cannot really object to what one might call the Recovery movement. It is of course well-intentioned, a bit happy-clappy; it emphasises the positive. You are not ill, but on a journey of recovery. Wellness is your goal. You can take control of your life and develop wellness strategies. People do not suffer from mental illness any more; they have mental health problems.

Orwell, again: 'Given, for instance, the word *good*, there was no need for such a word as *bad*, since the required meaning was equally well – indeed, better – expressed by the word *ungood*. All that was necessary, in any case where two words formed a natural pair of opposites, was to decide which one of them to suppress'.

No more illness. Just a question of being less well, more well, maybe even, or-well.

Thus, using a diagnosis like schizophrenia becomes by implication akin to sentencing someone to life imprisonment, without hope of remission. "Recovery" offers hope. Fair enough: no one wants to deprive the sick and suffering of hope.

It is all part of the contemporary climate of political correctness. Evasiveness, I prefer to call it: an extreme unwillingness to name or face up to the unpalatable. People are no longer blind, but visually impaired; no longer elderly, just older; no longer disabled, but less able; they no longer fail exams, merely experience delayed success. And if a hospital kills someone by mistake it is recorded as an SUI, a serious untoward incident.

Let us eliminate the negative, the judgemental, all that which tends to place people in categories. Stereotyping is *ungood* and some stereotyping is more *ungood* than others. Take black-and-minority-ethnic, for example – BMEs for short: that is good stereotyping, because it is associated with other obvious goods, like equality, diversity, respect and inclusion, *Rethink*'s core beliefs (annual report 2005/6) – and who could be so churlish as to question the value of any of these. What you have to be to qualify as BME we are never really told. For instance, is French ethnic? Are Syrians black? Do university-educated or wealthy Bangladeshis belong in the same category as illiterate peasants from Sylhet? And how is any of this relevant to anyone's affliction by or treatment for mental illness?

Orwell, again: speaking of the tendency in Newspeak to use abbreviations (particularly noticeable in totalitarian organisations and countries, he observes) like *Comintern*, *Gestapo*, *Agitprop*, he says this was done deliberately because 'in thus abbreviating a name one narrowed and subtly altered its meaning, cutting out most of the associations that would otherwise cling to it'. Is not the effect of using acronyms like BMEs rather similar? '*Comintern* is a word that can be uttered almost without taking thought.' For *Comintern* substitute BMEs: you do not stop to think about Syrians or Italians or Bangladeshi peasants.

Why the language of political correctness should be applied to mental illness in this way and not, say, to more obviously pathological conditions like heart disease, I am not sure, unless it is that all mental illness is indeed seen in the light of "some kind of mental health problem", a response in effect to life experiences: a social or existential problem, not a medical one. There is a very marked difference in the way the people receiving and the people administering treatment for, say, kidney disease, cancer, ankle sprains and coughs view what is happening between them and the way in which those who receive treatment for mental illness view their treatment. In the former case the relationship is consensual, the patient trusting in both the expertise and the well-disposedness of his doctor. In the latter the doctor's intervention is often experienced as hostile by the patient and almost invariably presented as hostile by both the caring professions and the organisations that purport to speak for the mentally ill.

The "ethos of recovery", *Rethink* tells us, is driven by the survivor/user movement. The very name survivor points to what their attitude to treatment is. And one should not forget that it is not many years since even *MIND* opposed the use of antipsychotic medication, while *Rethink* is always making much of its successful opposition to the government's attempt to incorporate some kind of compulsory treatment order in its new mental health legislation. This is partly knee-jerk defence of our ancient English liberties (selective, generally: what about the poor smokers?) and partly a consequence of the continuing tendency to view psychiatry as a repressive tool for state and society to use against its dissenting or non-conforming citizens. How else can one explain the extraordinary intervention by Paul Farmer, then a spokesman for *Rethink*, on a Channel Four news programme in November 2005 in which he attacked the use of "sections" – the power under the Mental Health Act to detain people against their will, a power that has many times saved the lives of our children – against a backdrop, presumably designed by Channel Four, consisting of menacing closed doors, the effect of which, presumably desired, was to imply that compulsory treatment under the Mental Health Act was not much different from Soviet

Russian use of psychiatric hospitals for disposing of the politically tiresome.

Rethink justifies its positions on the grounds that it is responding to "users'" wishes, without ever making clear who those "users" are, whether they are what one might call the walking wounded or the seriously ill. It does not take much imagination to guess what the results of a straw poll on a psychiatric ward would throw up: do you like taking medication, would you rather not be here, do you enjoy the lack of privacy, being shut up with a lot of other loonies, do you like being thought of as mad?

Doctors and scientists have no difficulty in calling spades spades; in fact it would be difficult to see how you could conduct research or prescribe a treatment if you could not bring yourself to name the problem you were investigating or make a diagnosis. It is the social services and charity bureaucrats who cannot bring themselves to name names and speak plain English. This contrast in approach was starkly evident in the speeches made at the Annual General Meeting of the old National Schizophrenia Fellowship at which the change of name to *Rethink* was announced: Professor Robin Murray of the Institute of Psychiatry and one of the most eminent researchers in schizophrenia in the land and himself a consultant psychiatrist, spoke all the time of schizophrenia in his address, while the then Chief Executive of *NSF/Rethink* and the driving force behind this change rehearsed the organisation's achievements without a single mention of the word.

Might it not just be possible that doctors, even allowing for the fact that psychiatry is still a relatively inexact science, are committed to making people better and may actually know a thing or two? The "iatrogenic" letter-writer quoted earlier sneered that the medical profession's 'expert power is embedded in conservative orthodoxies'. Would not you rather fly in an aircraft constructed according to the conservative orthodoxies of the engineering profession?

Does any of this matter? Well, yes, it does. For putting about the idea that doctors are somehow malign or incompetent, not to say both, hardly contributes to establishing a helpful therapeutic relationship between treater and treated. And that cannot be to anyone's advantage, particularly when dealing with an illness one of whose most notorious symptoms is a refusal to recognise that one is ill and needs treatment.

And there is a new element in this anti-psychiatry cocktail: race. *Rethink*, needless to say, holds "core beliefs on inclusion, respect, diversity and equality" (annual report 2005/6); every questionnaire comes accompanied by a diversity monitoring form. Lee Jasper, before his fall from grace as Ken Livingstone's adviser on "equalities", was promoting a campaign accusing British psychiatry of being "institutionally racist". The accusation appears to rest on the fact that there is a higher rate of diagnosis for schizophrenia among people of Afro-Caribbean origin living in the UK than among the native population. I attended a debate on this issue at the Maudsley Hospital in December 2006, where Lee Jasper and a Ghanaian psychiatrist spoke for the motion that psychiatry in Britain was institutionally racist while Dr Swaran Singh, an Indian psychiatrist, and Professor Robin Murray of the Maudsley spoke against. They based their case on various statistical studies which show that migrant communities, regardless of where they have emigrated from and where they have ended up, show significantly greater vulnerability to mental illness than indigenous populations, for what, one would have thought, pretty commonsensical reasons. (Rather in the same way that urban populations show a greater vulnerability than rural ones.) But no, in the current climate of multi-cultural sensitivity, we have to go for race as the explanation.

It was instructive to watch Lee Jasper at work. When he took the platform, I had the strong impression that he had not prepared what he was going to say. He is a factory gate politician. You could see him winding himself up to full rhetorical momentum, with references to slavery and the *SS Windrush*, the ship that brought the first West Indian workers to Britain in 1950. What the relevance of this might be to racism in psychiatry was not clear. It was part of a performance designed to rouse the rabble, to stir his listeners into responding with a vote by acclamation.

But when you think about it, how could an institution be racist, unless its constitution embodies overtly racist provisions?

Individuals, maybe, but an institution? And how would racism manifest itself in psychiatry, unless the practice of it were based on stated theories about the relation between race and certain conditions for which the only evidence was racial difference? And even then it would have to be shown to be discriminatory in negative ways, in ways that led to unjust treatment. It is difficult to see why even individual psychiatrists with racist beliefs would make life harder for themselves by handing out diagnoses of schizophrenia unnecessarily, thereby overpopulating their wards with stroppy and recalcitrant patients. Surely being racist implies malevolent intent?

And there you would be wrong. For here is another word whose meaning has been altered to suit a particular politics. Institutional racism apparently is what happens when "...forces, social arrangements, institutions, structures, policies, precedents and systems of social relations... operate to deprive certain racially identified categories of equality". And you can be guilty of racism without knowing it and without intending it; intent is no longer a requirement. If I say you are racist, then you are. Rather as with Recovery: evidence not required: if I say I am recovered, then I am.

Scientists with solid reputations like Professor Murray and Dr Singh say that racism does not explain the higher apparent incidence of schizophrenia in some immigrant populations. Any visitor to big city psychiatric wards can see for himself that a high proportion of staff are black. Furthermore, something like 45% of psychiatrists practising in the UK are of non-European origin: facts, one would have thought, which do not sit comfortably with accusations of racism?

Rethink has signed up to this notion with enthusiasm. "There is a lot of evidence about institutional racism in mental health services," Jane Harris, Head of Campaigns and Media, told me in a letter of Nov 8th 2007, although she did not explain what it was.

Racism is an accusation. It is certainly intended as such by the likes of Lee Jasper. It is bad news. It is something one would not be proud of. It is something you can be prosecuted for. If there is no intent to deprive anyone of equal treatment on racial grounds, is it fair to accuse a person, let alone an institution, of racism?

Might it not be that the institutions in a country like this, indeed in any country developed enough to have institutions like health services and universities, have developed, were shaped, to suit the needs, values and beliefs of the people living in those countries during the period of the development of these institutions? Might not this be the reason why the new boy on the block, the immigrant recently arrived, especially when he comes from a country where higher education is almost unknown, where corruption is endemic, where social relations are organised along clannish and partisan rather than rational and civic lines, might not this be the explanation for any mismatch between his expectations, beliefs and values and those of the host community? Cultural misunderstanding, in other words, and not racism.

Promoting the notion that the mental health services are racist merely serves to undermine further the crucial therapeutic relationship between doctor and patient. And if the evidence for such a claim is spurious, it is downright irresponsible.

*

A number of years have now elapsed since *Rethink* decreed that stigma, fear, prejudice and ignorance were the main problems facing people suffering from "mental health problems" in this country. Have its activities made one iota of difference to the experience of people ill with schizophrenia? Have they made any difference to the problem of the over-occupancy of hospital beds? To the stock of available accommodation? To the supervision of people discharged from hospital? To ensuring that they are taking their medication, eating properly, looking after themselves, washing, doing the laundry, getting the benefits they are entitled to? Have they contributed anything to simplifying and smoothing out any of the complexities and inconsistencies in the benefits system – which are already hard enough for someone without mental health problems to negotiate? Have they contributed anything to making it easier for a father, a mother, a sister, to intervene on behalf of a sick relative, to obtain or provide any kind of information without running up against the obsession with consent, privacy, confidentiality, data protection, rights, that characterises every branch of officialdom? No, no, and again no, is the answer to all these questions. And these are precisely the areas in which people need help.

In 2007 *Rethink*, in partnership with *MIND*, won a Lottery grant of £16 million to fight stigma and discrimination. I have in front of me its *Executive Summary* (whatever that is) of the *Rethink* Anti-Discrimination Site (RAS) Pilot Evaluation. This is its own evaluation of the success of a dry-run for its campaign against stigma: the erection in Norwich in 2006 of a statue of Winston Churchill in a straitjacket, intended to show how mental illness (Churchill's "black dog" depressions) need not be an impediment to worldly success. 'Our campaign,' it announces, 'had a significant impact on the public's awareness of, and attitudes towards, people with mental ill health.'

No indication is given of how their results were arrived at or how big the sample of people questioned was. Among other things they tell us, 'We used adverts on local buses and radio with strong messaging and branding.' For example: 'Call me mad because I believe Norwich City will get promoted. Not because I have schizophrenia,' and 'Think I'm strange because I like homework. Not because I have a mental illness.'

I telephoned Norwich Tourist Information Office while all this was going on; they said they had never heard of any such campaign nor indeed of any statue of Winston Churchill in a straitjacket. I harbour a suspicion that the Lottery's £16 million might yield better results invested in Professor Murray's research programmes or indeed *Rethink*'s ambition to raise the standards of its "style and presentation" to those of the "Plain English Campaign".

*

The autumn 2007 issue of *Rethink*'s magazine *Your Voice* carried an article, "The hijacking of schizophrenia", by its deputy editor, Terry Hammond, who also has a son suffering from schizophrenia.

Schizophrenia, he writes, 'is fast becoming "the neglected illness" and all this is happening in the name of "recovery" – "empowerment" – "independence"...I believe there is *no comparison between the life-changing effects caused by schizophrenia and other forms of mental illness* (my emphasis)...Most people who develop schizophrenia do not go on to live "normal" lives. Most are unable to work. Few get married or successfully socially integrate nor do they become prime ministers, spin doctors, comic geniuses or award-winning actors!' He goes on to say that 'one of the key reasons, in my view, why society is failing to understand schizophrenia as an illness, is because too many policy makers and politicians have been taken in by the ideological claptrap which has been preached over the years by the mental health "extremists"... you mustn't mention the word "illness". "It's all the fault of the medical system", or that "day centres are institutional and regressive". Clichés rule, ok – empowerment, independence, normalisation, recovery: all worthy aspirations, yes, but in the hands of politicians and Primary Care Trusts, they are simply excuses for delivering community care on the cheap... It is not just the extremists who are to blame, it is also a small group of service users who have had the ear of the government and have misrepresented the needs of people with schizophrenia. Why? Because most of those who are campaigning at this level are individuals with depressive and anxiety disorders – not schizophrenia.'

I am used to my contributions to this debate being ignored; for I obviously belong to the lunatic fringe. It was interesting, however, to see the response to Terry Hammond, a *Rethink* employee, after all. Clearly he touched a raw nerve, for an inordinate amount of space was given to replies by other staff members refuting his arguments. Here is just one, by the Director of Service Improvement, the gist of it highlighted thus: 'I would suggest that in *Rethink* services a recovery ethos is tangible and evidenced in practice' .

Quite so!

Epilogue

In November 2006 *The Observer* published an article I had written in which I touched on many of the things I have written about in this book. It prompted a letter, sent care of the paper, from a young woman who had been a friend of my son's at university: it was the most touching and, to me, most precious response I have received from anyone in the long years of this illness.

It is so easy in all the mess and frustration, anguish and humiliation, to forget how very different things once were, how bright and full of hope, how special this person whose agonies you have watched over with such weary anxiety once was. She said: 'My stomach lurched when I read this article... Jeremy really shone at university. So charismatic, cool, handsome and intelligent. He was always such a pleasure to be with and had impeccable musical taste. I recall spending a lot of time lounging on his bed listening to some obscure and totally outrageous funk track or other. He had a picture on his wall of a hard core soul brother riding on the back of a dolphin... I even recognise the jumper he is wearing in *The Observer* picture as he used to wear it a lot in Edinburgh!

'I met you once. You and Jeremy accompanied Paul and me to a Paul Brady concert. I remember being outraged as the three of you got bored halfway through and decamped to the bar...

'Jeremy was so proud of you and talked a lot about your work. He made us laugh with stories of fact-finding missions on your behalf where he would have to spend hours researching tedious matters like bike hire charges instead of chasing girls and drinking beer in the sun as he would have preferred...

'... I wanted you to know that I read it and have thought a lot about your family today. Please tell Jeremy that B sends her love.'

*

Jeremy was forty-two last Sunday. I made him a cake again – 'like a cliff of chocolate, Dad' – and took it over. His mother was there and his girlfriend. He was washed and brushed and had on a new pair of trousers and his smart black shoes that only rarely get an airing. His hair, thinning on his high forehead, waved elegantly back over his ears. His eyes were clear. With his glasses on the end of his nose he looked like a benign and handsome professor. We had a glass or two of champagne. Autumn sunlight poured in his window...

He is much better than he has ever been before. "Ftoo, ftoo!" as the Greeks say and toss salt over their shoulders as a precautionary measure against the evil eye. I could not say with any certainty how long this relative wellness – because it is relative – might last. It is due, I think, to two things. One is the regular medication: he has been regularly medicated for more than three years now and that goes a long way towards controlling the psychotic symptoms. He does still hear voices and they do still seem to get associated with neighbours. I remain unclear about their precise status. Sometimes he does seem to understand that while he may experience them as coming from an external source they are actually "inner speech". At other times I am not so sure. But then it may be that when he complains of the neighbours' voices that is indeed what he is hearing. After all you can hear neighbours' voices in a block of flats. Perhaps, living alone as he does, he is particularly sensitive to extraneous sound. I am; I have a very low tolerance of noise that is not of my choosing. Maybe he has inherited that from me. I worry about his voices because I fear the trouble they might get him into. Perhaps I should not.

The other important factor that contributes to his being so much better is his own greater wisdom. He has learnt to manage his illness much better. He has much more insight, as they like to say. He will talk about being schizophrenic. He is proud of having a little circle of friends in the area where he lives and can say of them quite openly that they have all got mental health problems, including himself in this general category. His social skills, you might think, still leave something to be desired but he is able to show some understanding of other people's reactions and feelings; he can be patient, he will sit in a strange café without fleeing at the arrival of strangers at the next table, he does travel on the bus, he does manage to do some shopping. He asks me how I am when he rings up, he asks after my wife. He tells me how much he loves me and thanks me for things I have done for him. He apologises for being rude or difficult or morose. 'If I seem to crack sometimes, Dad, it is not me, it's the schizophrenia.'

It may seem a rather curious thing to say but I think the surest measure of how much things have improved is his willingness to go to the dentist. There you are, trapped in a chair, at the mercy of a stranger, submitting to the infliction of pain, another stranger in the person of the nurse fussing around you... If that is not a situation likely to bring on an attack of extreme paranoia I do not know what is. Yet he makes his appointments and, more importantly, keeps them. As he had not been near a dentist for the best part of twenty years, there have been rather a lot of them, which makes the achievement all the more impressive. I think it is also a considerable tribute to the kindness, good nature and humanity of the dentist. He is my dentist too and I am deeply grateful to him.

Perhaps age too plays a role. The fury that drives a young man in his twenties has abated, the testosterone does not rage quite as madly. You can begin to stand back with a bit of objectivity from your own life. I am often surprised by how much my son seems to have reflected on his difficult and unusual experience. His intellect seems to have been restored, repaired, too. Whether it is the regular medication or the wisdom gained I do not know, but there has been a definitive recovery of cognitive ability.

To the uninitiated these may seem pathetically small and trivial grounds for rejoicing – and more than likely precariously gained at that. I think of what must have been my mother's joy when my father, after his second dose of ECT treatment, saw her, recognised her and smiled and knew his name again. He had come back, returned, re-inhabited his mortal human form, could be communicated with again in normal everyday banalities: 'Would you like a boiled egg for breakfast?'

The small signs that someone is returning from the more desolate shores of schizophrenia are similarly grounds for rejoicing. A friend who knows my son told me the other day that he had seen him in the street a couple of times and commented that he looked perfectly normal: you would not have known there was anything wrong with him. I was pathetically flattered and grateful!

'I don't believe it's a deteriorating disease, and I don't see this inevitable progression that people talk about. If you treat patients enthusiastically and appropriately at onset, then some of them will make a good recovery...' Professor Murray told the Schizophrenia Research Forum in his 2005 interview.

"Enthusiastically.." Now there is the rub. What might not have happened if our generation of children had been treated enthusiastically at onset, if someone had made a committed, warm-hearted attempt to engage with them, hear what they had to say, instead of subjecting them to what Prof Murray calls "a kind of veterinary medicine".

Speaking of psychiatry, the interviewer said to Prof Murray: 'Compared to other arms of medicine, expectations somehow seem low. Do you agree?' Prof Murray replied that psychiatry 'has been starved of resources. The fault may lie partly with us because we haven't shouted loud enough about the neglect of the mentally ill, but it mainly lies with the rest of society who don't care about people with schizophrenia. Treating the mentally ill has not had the priority it deserves'.

Yesterday I gave Jeremy a lift to the dentist to have a tooth pulled. While he was there his girlfriend phoned to say that a man in the bed-and-breakfast accommodation where she is living was taking her socks from the communal laundry and using them for masturbating. She has a long history of mental illness too. She used to have a council flat. It was "invaded" by a gang of young black drug dealers who inveigled a key out of her, came and went as they pleased and threatened her with violence if she were to tell anyone. Eventually the social services moved her, into this bed-and-breakfast hotel. She has been there several months already. To move back into a flat of her own she has to go through the Council's bidding procedure; she is waiting for them to give her the appropriate number of points so she can start bidding again. She has a daughter and a baby grand-daughter. Why is she in bed-and-breakfast accommodation? Whose need is greater than hers? She had to wait long enough to be rescued from the youths who had invaded the home where she brought up her daughter. Why did she have to wait so long? She has no one to fight her corner, no one to come to her aid when subjected to harassment by a strange man. Why not? Is this a civilised way of treating some of our most vulnerable fellow beings?

Three days ago I was walking past Keats's house in the rain. I had an umbrella up. I spotted a man about my son's age coming towards me. He was someone I have often seen on the psychiatric wards, a well-spoken, educated man. He is always begging on the streets in this neighbourhood. I hid under my umbrella so he could not see my face. Sure enough, from under the rim of the umbrella, I saw his ragged trouser bottoms crossing the street towards me. 'Billy,' I said, raising the brolly, 'why are you begging still? Why aren't you getting your benefits?'

This time he told me he had just come from the hospital where he had been for some "assessments". I do not know whether it was true. Last time he told me he had been evicted. Again I do not know if it was true. 'Can you give me a pound, Mr Salmon?' 'Billy,' I said, 'no, I am not going to give you a pound. I'm always giving you pounds.'

Does he have a home? Is he getting any benefits? Does he have a social worker or a CPN? Does he have a Care Plan and a Care Co-ordinator? Is anybody looking after him? Perhaps wandering the streets begging is part of his well-being agenda, a stage in his recovery journey?

My son is doing okay – at the moment. Yet even so when his light bulbs go he does not replace them. He would live in darkness if I were not there. He does not starve, but he has not had what my mother would have considered a proper balanced meal in twenty years. He tidies up his flat, occasionally, perfunctorily and unsystematically. I do not know how long it would be before it became a health hazard if his mother and I were not around. Thank God he has got a flat, of his own: not some melancholy, impersonal, institutional bedsit or a grotty room in a "hotel" designed deliberately to exploit the poorest of the poor being housed by the DSS.

If schizophrenia is indeed caused by the collision of a number of "susceptibility genes" and "a toxic social environment", then it would seem somewhat self-defeating to allow schizophrenic patients to be exposed to such obviously toxic environmental factors as part of their treatment.

If my son is as well as he is, it is not because anyone has empowered him or mapped out any flexible pathways or socially included him or waved him off like a latter-day Dick Whittington on a self-directed journey of recovery with a packet of clichés wrapped in a kerchief on the end of pole. He can take most of the credit himself. It is largely his own achievement, more in spite of rather than thanks to any system put in place by the state or the agencies to which it passes on or, rather, shrugs off, responsibility.

He has just phoned. 'Hello, how are you this morning?'

'I'm okay, thank you, young man.'

'I'm glad to hear that, old man. How's the age difference this morning?'

'Pretty much the same as yesterday, I think.'

'It won't be if you go on riding your bike up East Hill at your age.'

'I went to the gym in the end.'

'Oh yes, you said. Well, I feel pretty good today. I had a bit of a downer last night. I went to the W and had half a pint of Guinness. I ordered a pint but I could not...'

'Do it by halves,' I said, fussing as usual. 'They charge so much, you don't want to leave half.'

'I know. Anyway, it didn't work and I went home and had a BLT and didn't feel good.'

'Probably because the BLT wasn't enough.'

'No, you're right.'

'Have you done the washing up?'

'No, I haven't,' he said.

'There was so much of it you couldn't do any cooking anyway. I'll come over and give you a hand tomorrow.'

'That's good. It'll probably be done. If you're coming over that will give me a spur to do it.'

And so it goes on. We are entering our twenty-first year. Maybe he will want to see me tomorrow, maybe he won't. It just remains to stay alive as long as possible.

THE END

About The Author

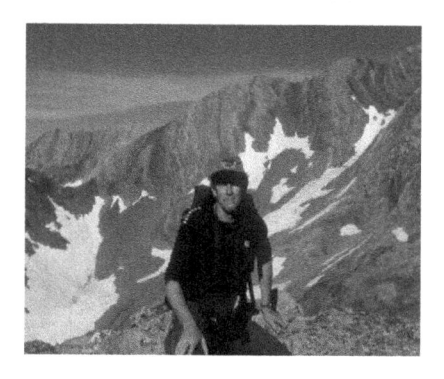

Tim Salmon is the author of several books about Greece, including a cook book, a walker's guide to the mountains and *The Unwritten Places,* an account of his travels in the Pindos range. He was one of the original authors of *The Rough Guide to France* and *The Rough Guide to Paris*. For more than thirty years, he has contributed to national newspapers and magazines such as *The Guardian, Independent, Telegraph, The Times, Time Out* and *Country Life*.

An indefatigable traveller, Tim's adventures have included trips to the mountains of Tajikistan, walking the length of France (described in *On Foot Across France: Dunkirk to the Pyrenees*) and making a documentary for Greek TV about transhumant shepherds moving their flocks from the mountains of the north to their winter pastures in the lowlands. In 2010, Tim appeared on BBC Radio 4's *All In The Mind* to talk about schizophrenia, prompting a huge public response.

Website: TimSalmon.org

Acknowledgements

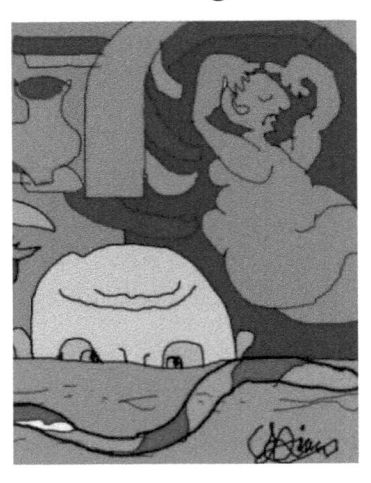

I'd like particularly to thank and pay to tribute to my friend, Adam Grieve. He is a talented artist who has kindly contributed one of his images for us to use as the cover of this book. He is a very courageous man who has kept up his work as a painter and sculptor while himself battling for many years against the difficulties and distress caused by schizophrenia.

http://adamgrieve.com

Reader Resources

Sane: http://www.sane.org.uk/
Rethink: http://www.rethink.org/

To keep up to date with all Tim Salmon news, events and new titles join the Tim Salmon mailing list
http://eepurl.com/CWOGL
(All email details are securely managed at Mailchimp.com and are never shared with third parties.)

If this book has lived up to your expectations, please would you consider leaving a review? Amazon.com for US or Amazon.co.uk for UK? A couple of lines is plenty. It really makes all the difference to us small independent publishers who rely on word of mouth to get our books known. Thank you!

http://blackbird-books.com
Twitter: @blackbirdebooks
Email: blackbird.digibooks@gmail.com

We publish rights-reverted titles by established quality authors alongside exciting new talent.

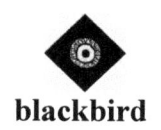

blackbird